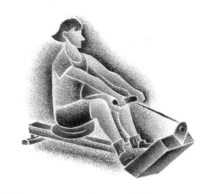

Health And Healing
The Natural Way

EXERCISE AND YOUR HEALTH

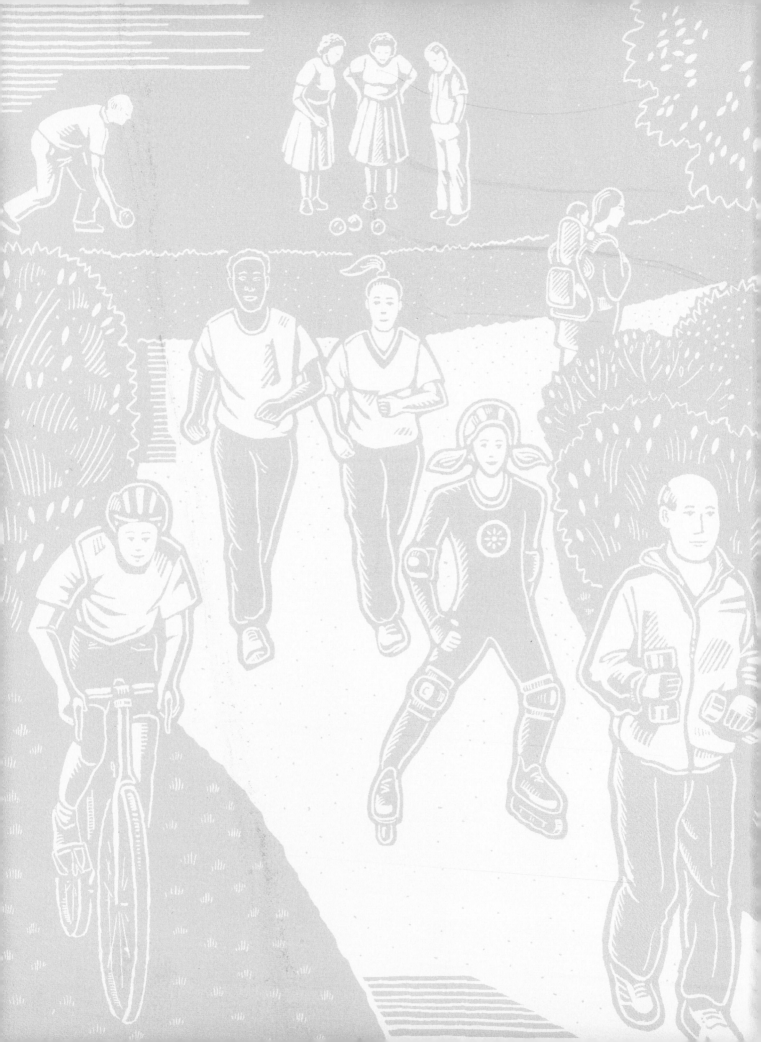

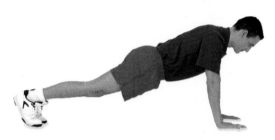

HEALTH AND HEALING
THE NATURAL WAY

EXERCISE AND YOUR HEALTH

Reader's
Digest

PUBLISHED BY

THE READER'S DIGEST ASSOCIATION, INC.

PLEASANTVILLE, NEW YORK / MONTREAL

A READER'S DIGEST BOOK
Produced by
Carroll & Brown Limited, London

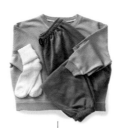

CARROLL & BROWN

Publishing Director Denis Kennedy
Art Director Chrissie Lloyd

Managing Editor Sandra Rigby
Managing Art Editor Tracy Timson

Project Coordinator Laura Price

Editor Richard Emerson

Design Mercedes Morgan,
Rachel Goldsmith, Simon Daley

Photographers Jules Selmes, David Murray

Production Wendy Rogers, Karen Kloot

Computer Management John Clifford, Paul Stradling

Copyright © 2000 The Reader's Digest Association, Inc.
Copyright © 2000 The Reader's Digest Association (Canada) Ltd.
Copyright © 2000 Reader's Digest Association Far East Ltd.
Philippine Copyright © 2000 Reader's Digest Association Far East Ltd.

Printed in the United States of America

Library of Congress Cataloging in Publication Data

Exercise and Your Health / Reader's Digest.
        p. cm. — (Health and healing the natural way)
    ISBN 0-7621-0265-9
    1.Exercise—health aspects. 2. Health—Physiological
aspects. I. Reader's Digest Association.   II. Series.
RA781 .E892 2000
613.7'1 —dc21
                                        99-054712

The information in this book is for reference only;
it is not intended as a substitute for a doctor's diagnosis and care.
The editors urge anyone with continuing medical problems
or symptoms to consult a doctor.

CONSULTANTS

Bob Smith MA, BEd Hons, Cert Ed
*Department of Physical Education, Sports Science and
Recreation Management, Loughborough University*

Dr. Amanda Roberts MB, BChir

CONTRIBUTORS

Professor Ron Maughan BSc, PhD
Professor of Human Physiology

Dr. Lorraine Cale BSc, MSc, PhD
Lecturer in Physical Education

Dr. Briony Thomas BSc, PhD, SRD, *Nutritionist*

Tim Cable PhD, *Reader in Exercise Physiology*

Penny Hunking SRD, *Accredited Sports Dietitian*

Rozalind Gruben Prof AHSI, RSA
Health and Fitness Consultant

Kelly Hosking BEd Hons, *Fitness Consultant*

Fiona Hayes, *Fitness Consultant*

READER'S DIGEST PROJECT STAFF

Series Editor Gayla Visalli
Editorial Director, Health & Medicine Wayne Kalyn
Design Director Barbara Rietschel
Production Technology Manager Douglas A. Croll
Editorial Manager Christine R. Guido
Art Production Coordinator Jennifer R. Tokarski

READER'S DIGEST ILLUSTRATED REFERENCE BOOKS, U.S.

Editor-in-Chief Christopher Cavanagh
Art Director Joan Mazzeo
Operations Manager William J. Cassidy

READER'S DIGEST BOOKS & HOME ENTERTAINMENT, CANADA

Vice President and Editorial Director Deirdre Gilbert
Managing Editor Philomena Rutherford
Art Director John McGuffie

Address any comments about *Exercise and Your Health* to
Editor in Chief, U.S. Illustrated Reference Books,
Pleasantville, NY 10570

Exercise and Your Health

More and more people today are choosing to take greater responsibility for their own health rather than relying on their doctor to step in with a cure when something goes wrong. It is now recognized that we can influence our health by making certain improvements in lifestyle—eating better, doing more exercise, and taking measures to reduce stress, for example. People are also becoming increasingly aware that there are other healing methods—some new, others ancient—that can help prevent illness or be used as complements to orthodox medicine.

The series *Health and Healing the Natural Way,* which provides clear, comprehensive, straightforward, and encouraging information and advice about methods of improving health, can help you make informed health choices. The series explains the many different natural therapies now available, including aromatherapy, herbalism, acupressure, and a number of others, as well as the circumstances in which they may be of benefit when used in conjunction with conventional medicine.

For people who have led essentially sedentary lives up to now or who are moderately active but want to increase their fitness levels, establishing a regular exercise routine or a more intensive one can seem daunting. However, everyone can incorporate healthy exercise into their daily lives with surprisingly little effort and disruption. *Exercise and Your Health* shows you ways you can become fitter with just a few alterations in your lifestyle; it's not necessary to establish a grueling training routine. The book explains how to build up exercise levels gradually and safely and assess your progress along the way. In return for the effort, major health benefits will accrue, such as less illness, increased stamina and strength, and a more positive outlook. You may discover not only how enjoyable exercise can be but also how easily it becomes a part of your life—and how much you will miss it if you skip a few days.

CONTENTS

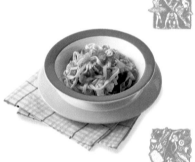
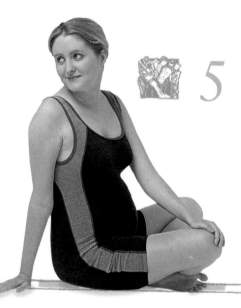
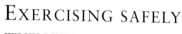

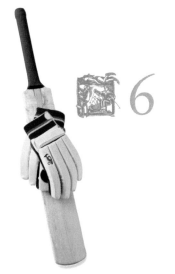

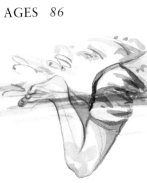

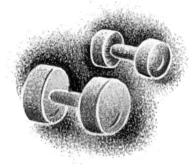

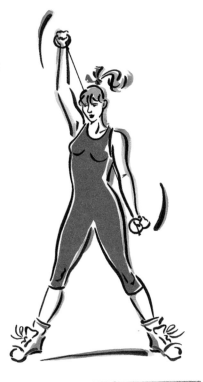

FIT FOR LIFE

Doing exercise that you enjoy can be not only a satisfying pastime but also an opportunity to greatly enhance your quality of life.

Most of us are aware of how exercise can improve health but may still find it difficult to overcome entrenched habits and attitudes to make the change toward a more active lifestyle. Yet the process needn't be intimidating nor a chore. There are plenty of ways to exercise that are fun and rewarding in their own right. For example, activities like team sports and dancing are great ways to meet new people and socialize with friends, as well as to become fit. Exercise can also be a means of relieving stress in your daily life. Yoga and t'ai chi, for instance, are calming and relaxing and also build strength and flexibility.

Exercise need not involve long sessions of physical activity. Short workouts three or four times a day, which most people can easily fit into an average schedule, can be just as effective. A study from the University of Pittsburgh found the same level of fitness benefit for women who did 10 minutes of exercise four times a day as for those who did 40-minute sessions once a day. But many people still aren't getting enough exercise, even though in recent years there has been much focus on the link between fitness and health.

THE DECLINE OF EXERCISE

For past generations physical effort was an inescapable part of daily life. Until early in the 20th century, most men and many women worked in physically demanding manual trades, while for the majority of women, housework and child rearing, without the benefit of labor-saving devices was a constant round of physical work. Even leisure periods were likely to involve some effort. Dancing was one of the most popular pastimes for all ages, and most people expected to walk at least part of the way to social events or work. The average person's basic calorie intake has actually altered little over the past 100 years, yet obesity was not a major issue a century ago. One reason for the difference is that people in Western society have a more sedentary lifestyle today,

QUICK STEP TO FITNESS Being active does not necessarily mean being an athlete. Regular dancing sessions provide plenty of stamina-boosting exercise and offer lots of opportunities for socializing as well.

and the calories they consume are not burned up at the same rate in fueling physical activity. The advent of cars, television, and modern household appliances and the switch from manual labor to automated or clerical jobs have meant that most people are far less active than in the past. When someone who is used to low levels of activity attempts something more strenuous, such as running to catch a bus, the effort can lead to medical problems, from strains and sprains to heart attack and stroke.

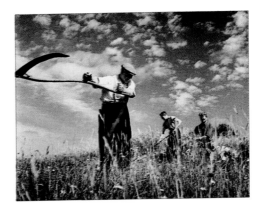

ALL WORK
In the past most people got enough daily exercise from their occupations, but now the majority have sedentary jobs.

EXERCISE AND HEALTH

While no one advocates a return to backbreaking manual labor and dawn-to-dusk household drudgery, health experts do feel that the pendulum has swung too far toward inactivity and that many people now have too little physical effort in their lives. Researchers are constantly finding new evidence of the health benefits that exercise provides. For example, it is known that sustained exercise, such as brisk walking, jogging, or cycling, that raises the pulse and breathing rate for at least 20 minutes three times a week can help protect the heart and circulatory system from the major killers of the developed world—heart and artery disease and stroke.

Regular exercise, provided it is not taken to extremes, also boosts the body's immune system, helping to guard against cancer and other diseases. Weight-bearing exercise can strengthen the bones and thus help prevent osteoporosis, the brittle-bone condition that afflicts many people in later life.

THE STRENGTH TO COPE
Weight training is not just about building bigger muscles; regular strength exercises can help you cope much better with everyday tasks, such as housework, gardening, and looking after children.

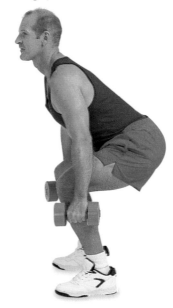

STRESS RELIEF

Exercise brings many important psychological benefits too. There is evidence that regular energetic exercise can increase the production of naturally occurring "feel-good" chemicals in the body, called endorphins, which help counteract anxiety and depression and enhance a feeling of general well-being. Exercise can also help alleviate another major scourge of the modern age—stress. Many people suffer levels of mental stress that are severe enough to cause physical symptoms, like sleeplessness and tension headaches, that may lead to serious disorders, such as ulcers and high blood pressure. In large part such problems result from the

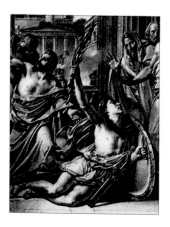

MARATHON MAN
According to legend, the Athenian Pheidippides ran nonstop from Marathon to Athens (some 26 miles) to announce a Greek victory and collapsed with the words "Rejoice, we conquer!"

FIND YOUR OWN LEVEL OF EXERCISE
You don't have to go to marathon levels to benefit from exercise. Many forms of physical activity, such as walking the dog every day or regularly gardening, can aid health and mental well-being and make daily tasks much easier to cope with.

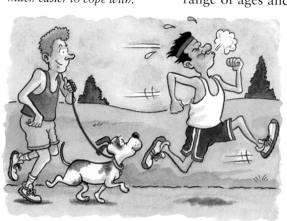

body's natural response to stress, which is to produce hormones that prepare it for a physical reaction. This "fight or flight" response helps us to counter physical threats—an essential attribute for our ancient ancestors, who were often faced with danger—but is less appropriate for dealing with modern causes of stress, such as relationship difficulties and work pressures. Exercise helps dissipate the stress hormones by channeling nervous energy into physical activity.

THE PEOPLE'S RACE

Once you become more active, you will be amazed by the exercise feats that become attainable. Most people think of the marathon as the supreme test of fitness, but with careful training more and more amateurs are now taking part in such races. The contest evolved from the achievement of the Greek messenger Pheidippides, who in 490 B.C. ran nonstop from Marathon to Athens—a little more than 26 miles, the distance run in today's marathons—to announce a decisive victory by the Athenians over the invading Persian army. The Battle of Marathon is now largely forgotten, but the race that commemorates that remarkable run is known worldwide.

The marathon was one of the main events at the first modern Olympic games, held in Athens in 1896. The first city marathon was held in Boston, Massachusets, in 1897 and comprised just 15 runners. A century later 40,000 runners took part in the Boston Marathon, and for many of them it was just one of several appearances they make at marathons in the world's major cities, including Tokyo, Paris, and the most famous venues, London and New York. For the majority the joy of the marathon is in completing the course, no matter how long it takes. Participants come from a wide range of ages and backgrounds. In a recent London Marathon, runners included a 73-year-old woman who had been sedentary until age 62 (see page 59).

Not all forms of exercise are as demanding as marathon running, of course. Whether the activity involves a competitive event, a keep-fit session at a gym, or a brisk walk in the countryside, there is a leisure pursuit to suit the fitness level, commitment, and personal interests of everyone. By far the most important issue is to find an activity that you enjoy and that you will be able to sustain.

EXERCISE FOR ALL AGES

It is vitally important to acquire the exercise habit at an early age. Young children are naturally energetic, but for older children and adolescents the attractions of such sedentary pastimes as television and computer games can prove a more powerful draw than active leisure pursuits. In addition, schools tend to place less emphasis on physical activities than in the past, and many parents now drive their children to school rather than letting them walk, which further reduces the opportunities for exercise. By helping children at an early age to find an activity that they can enjoy and encouraging them to continue with it, parents can ensure that their children reap the health benefits of exercise well into old age.

Exercise is not, of course, the sole province of the young. People of all ages and fitness levels can find active leisure pursuits that are both a source of enjoyment and an aid to better health. Swimming, for example, can be enjoyed at many levels and can be especially useful for elderly people, allowing them to exercise the limbs, heart, and lungs while the water provides support for weakened muscles and painful joints. Research shows that for sedentary people health benefits are achieved through even a modest increase in activity, such as a daily walk of 10 to 20 minutes.

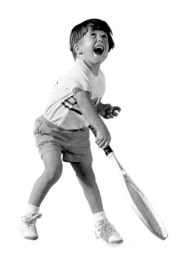

IMPORTANCE OF PLAYTIME
By encouraging young children to take part in physical games, you can aid their physical development and also promote hand and eye coordination.

KEEPING FIT AND HAVING FUN

For many people the primary purpose of an active leisure pursuit is to have fun, and keeping fit is a bonus. However, it has never been easier to find a sport or activity to suit an individual's interests, finances, and commitment. Most people are within easy traveling distance of a gym that offers a range of activities at a price they can afford. In addition, golf courses and health clubs are springing up at an ever-increasing rate, and many companies are providing exercise facilities on their premises or sponsoring their own sports teams.

Sports and exercise also provide important social opportunities; examples are the friendly outings of a walking group, the close bonding between badminton or tennis doubles partners, and the boisterous camaraderie of a soccer or rugby team. For many, such social interaction gives shape and purpose to their lives, while the support and encouragement of others enables them to push themselves farther than might otherwise have been possible.

VALUE FOR MONEY
Taking up a new sport may mean an initial investment in a few items of equipment and comfortable shoes. However, in the long term, exercise is one of the most economical forms of entertainment.

HOW TO USE THIS BOOK

The purpose of *EXERCISE AND YOUR HEALTH* is to encourage an active lifestyle and give advice on how to derive more enjoyment and greater health benefits from exercise. Chapter 1 looks at the effects of exercise on the body and shows how it can improve the quality of life—physically, mentally, and emotionally. In addition to bringing about physical changes that make it easier to carry out ordinary tasks, exercise can also improve such disorders as high blood pressure, arthritis, and asthma.

Chapter 2 covers the different types of exercise and explains what each one can help you achieve in terms of enhancing general fitness, boosting strength, and improving flexibility. It looks at the various components of a well-balanced fitness program and compares different activities to show what type of exercise each one provides.

The important link between exercise and diet is dealt with in Chapter 3. This section of the book examines the various roles that different nutrients play in exercise and fitness and shows how to plan your diet to make sure that you get the most out of an exercise regimen.

To monitor your progress during your fitness program, you need to know how to recognize and measure the improvements you are making. Chapter 4 looks at ways of testing your current physical status in regard to stamina, strength, and flexibility, and explains how to set attainable goals. Safety is a vital part of all sports and exercise, and Chapter 5 discusses the most suitable clothing to wear, how to avoid injury or other ill effects during exercise, and what to do if injury occurs. This chapter also looks at conditions that require extra caution in regard to exercise, such as pregnancy, illness, or the recovery period after surgery.

There is a wide range of leisure pursuits to choose from, and Chapter 6 aims to help you select the one that is right for you. It describes how to decide what your personal aspirations are, taking into account your age, budget, and level of commitment. Chapter 7 shows how you can incorporate more exercise into your daily life. It explains how to set up a home gym, describes exercises you can do both at home and at work, and suggests how you can involve the family and stay motivated. Finally, Chapter 8 describes what to look for in a health club, how to make the best use of the facilities, and how to choose a good instructor.

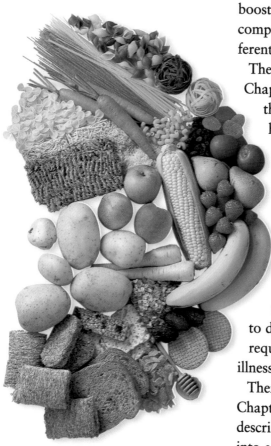

ENERGY FOR EXERCISE
Increasing your intake of whole grains, vegetables, and fruits while limiting your intake of fats and refined sugar and flour will give you more energy without leading to unwanted weight gain.

ARE YOU GETTING ENOUGH EXERCISE?

You may feel that you exercise enough each week by simply going for a leisurely stroll on a Sunday if the weather is fine. But if this is all the physical activity you get, it will not go very far toward protecting you against heart disease or preventing sprains and strains resulting from lifting a heavy object. A regular exercise regimen can make a big difference to your health and your quality of life.

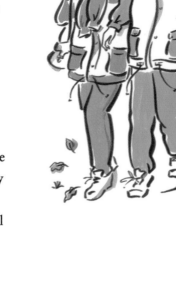

Q **IS IT A LONG TIME SINCE YOU EXERCISED? DO YOU FEEL THAT IT'S TOO LATE TO START NOW?**
It is never too late to begin some form of exercise program, no matter what your age or fitness level. In fact, research shows that for those who have been inactive for a long time, major health benefits can be achieved through a quite modest increase in exercise. Going for a leisurely walk each day for just 20 minutes, for example, can greatly reduce your risk of heart disease. As your fitness improves, you can increase your level of exertion to a brisk 20- to 40-minute walk three times a week. It will not be long before you feel a dramatic improvement in your general health and fitness. There are also many sport clubs that cater to senior members, allowing you to participate in a sport you may have enjoyed when you were younger and get back into the game at your own pace.

Q **DO YOU WANT TO GET FIT BUT DISLIKE THE IDEA OF JOGGING OR GOING TO THE GYM?**
A wide range of activities is within the reach of most people, so you are bound to find one or more pursuits that you can enjoy. Whether you are interested in walking or weight lifting, kayaking or karate, baseball or ballroom dancing, they all offer their own particular fitness benefits, as well as provide great opportunities to have fun. Some sports are best suited to those who prefer a mainly solitary activity, whereas others have a highly social element. Chapter 6 contains some suggestions, and you can ask at the library or a local sports or recreation center for a list of leisure activities offered in your neighborhood. It is also worth checking in the sports pages or advertisements in your local newspaper for groups in your area that are looking for new members. Try a few activities until you find ones that you like. You may discover that you need a little general fitness training as well. Chapters 7 and 8 have lots of exercise ideas for you to try.

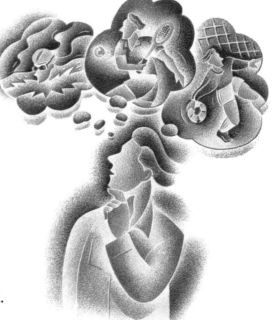

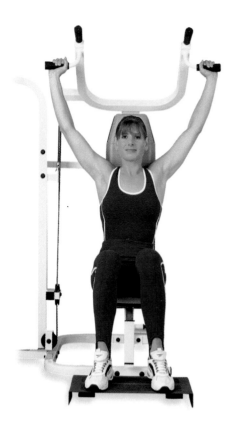

Q DO YOU FEEL THAT YOUR LIFE IS SIMPLY TOO BUSY FOR YOU TO FIT IN REGULAR EXERCISE?

With a little planning you can fit exercise into the busiest of schedules. For short journeys, walk instead of taking the car or a bus; you may find the trip is actually quicker on foot if you count the time you would have waited for the bus or spent parking the car. Make an effort twice a week to exercise during your lunch hour. Going for a brisk walk is simple enough, but if there is a gym or swimming pool nearby, you can fit in a 20- or 30-minute workout. This is time well spent, because regular exercise will sharpen your responses and make you more efficient at work. In the evening and on weekends, instead of watching television, go for a bicycle ride or a country ramble; if you have children, take them with you, and you can all enjoy the benefits of healthy exercise.

Q HAS YOUR CHRONIC BACKACHE OR JOINT PAIN BECOME AN EXCUSE TO AVOID EXERCISE?

Many people with chronic joint or muscle problems find that the mere thought of going to the gym or taking up jogging is just too painful to consider. In fact, many forms of exercise can be tailored to allow for injury, and they often help to relieve chronic pain. Some sports, such as aerobics, can be carried out in water to relieve pressure on joints and muscles. Others, like yoga, can be practiced in conjunction with a variety of sports to strengthen muscles and joints. It is important that you do not exacerbate a problem with the wrong sort of exercise, but there is no need to avoid exercise altogether. Check with a qualified trainer or fitness instructor, who can modify a workout to meet your needs.

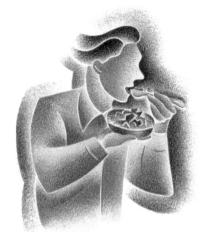

Q DO YOU HATE FEELING HUNGRY ALL THE TIME WHEN YOU DIET AND EXERCISE?

A common mistake that many people make is to think that the only way to lose weight is to starve yourself. If you are trying to follow a regular fitness program and at the same time stay on a very low-calorie diet, there is a risk that you will not get enough energy from your meals to meet your increased activity levels and will quickly become fatigued. In Chapter 3 we show that a planned, regular fitness program combined with a diet that is low in fat but high in protein and complex carbohydrates will provide all the energy you need and yet still help you lose weight. As you become fitter, your body will start to burn calories more efficiently, so you may end up eating more than you did before your diet yet still stay slim.

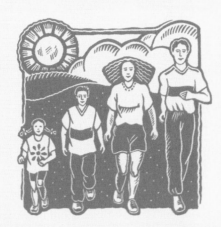

CHAPTER 1

HOW EXERCISE IMPROVES YOUR HEALTH

Exercise brings many benefits. It not only improves the physical condition of your body—your fitness, stamina, and strength—but also brings a feeling of mental well-being and increases self-confidence. Regular exercise can pave the way to a healthy, independent life well into old age.

WHY YOU SHOULD EXERCISE

One key to a healthy lifestyle, which will improve both physical and mental well-being, is to find a level of exercise that you find stimulating and can easily sustain on a regular basis.

The association between exercise and good health has been convincingly established over the years, and yet it is clear that from a health point of view the current lifestyle of the average person is still far from ideal. Even when people do exercise regularly, many of them do so at the lowest possible level; in the United States nearly 60 percent of people don't exercise enough to improve their health.

As information about the advantages of exercise has become widespread, more people have been taking up exercise on a recreational basis, but they don't necessarily keep it up. Every year thousands of people make New Year's resolutions to start working out in January, and by June at least half of them have given up. However, those who have abandoned exercise regimens can get started again if they re-examine the benefits.

HEALTH AND FITNESS

In general terms there are two clear benefits that can be obtained from regular exercise. The first is better health; the second is improvement in fitness. Although the concepts of health and fitness are often used as if they were interchangeable, there is a clear distinction between the two terms. The *Oxford English Dictionary* defines *health* as "soundness of body." More specifically, good health signifies the absence of illness and the efficient functioning of all the body's systems. Regular, sensible exercise can improve the efficiency of many of these systems, in particular the cardiovascular and respiratory. It can also boost the immune system, making those who exercise regularly less susceptible to colds and flu.

On the other hand, fitness means different things to different people. It can be broadly defined as the ability to perform everyday physical activities with vigor. The aim of the average person should be to achieve a level of fitness appropriate to his or her own needs. For some the basic level may mean being able to walk a reasonable distance without getting out of breath; for others it could be to play soccer in the park with their grandchildren. For a topnotch athlete fitness may mean pushing beyond present limits in competition with other athletes, the record books, or the elements.

Low levels of fitness are now recognized as a serious problem—perhaps the leading risk to general health—and are particularly linked to a susceptibility to cardiovascular diseases. The Framingham study, which began in Massachusetts in 1948, lasted more than 40 years, and involved 5,000 people, provided powerful evidence of this. The results of the study confirmed that

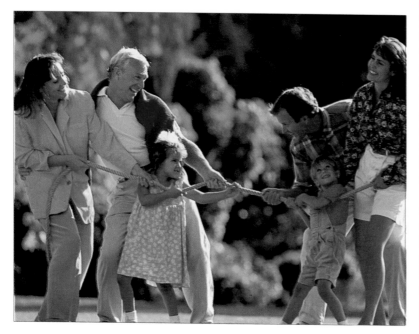

FAMILY EXERCISE
Simple games like tug-of-war, which can be enjoyed outdoors anywhere, encourage the whole family to include more healthy physical activities in their day.

people with very low levels of activity were over five times more likely to die from heart disease than those who incorporated moderate levels of exercise into their daily lives.

Mental and emotional fitness

The same arguments apply to mental and emotional fitness as to physical condition; it is not enough simply to be free of specific disorders. Just as exercise produces direct benefits to physical health, it also improves emotional and psychological well-being. Perhaps one of the most important benefits of exercise is its effectiveness in reducing stress, the long-term negative results of which are now well established.

A HEALTHY LIFESTYLE

Exercise plays an important part in a healthy lifestyle. When you exercise, you burn up energy and are less apt to put on weight. You also build strength, stamina, and muscle tone, gain confidence, and reduce stress, in addition to other important health benefits.

The case for regular exercise seems overwhelmingly convincing, yet the trend in recent years has been toward a less active lifestyle. In particular, children now spend more time in sedentary pursuits, like watching television, than in activities involving

HEALTH OF A NATION

More than 50 percent of adult North Americans are overweight, and almost one in four people of all ages is obese. Although poor eating habits have some bearing on these alarming statistics, inadequate exercise is also considered a major culprit. In the United States some 25 percent of the population are sedentary, while in Canada 8 percent participate in no regular exercise and as many as 38 percent of adults are inactice in their leisure time.

physical exercise. If this trend continues, it is likely to lead to serious health problems in the future. Yet exercise opportunities are more accessible than ever, with gyms, health clubs, and community exercise facilities now widely available. Even for people who cannot easily attend organized exercise sessions, the possibilities for increasing their level of physical activity are all around. And those who have rediscovered the physical potential of their bodies can attest to the health benefits and feelings of well-being that physical fitness brings.

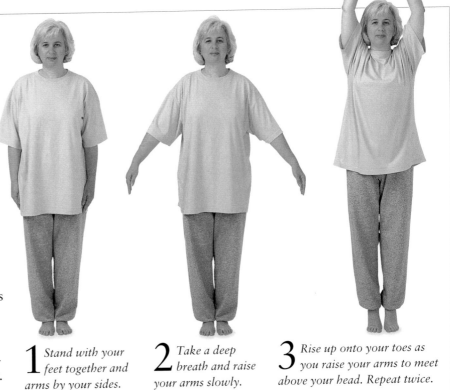

SIMPLE STRESS RELIEF

Regular exercise not only conditions and strengthens the body and improves fitness but also provides relief from many of life's everyday stresses.

Constant stress can lead to a range of specific diseases and illnesses, as well as contribute to negative emotional states like depression. Exercise provides an excellent release for the nervous tension produced by stress and helps you cope more effectively with everyday events.

The simple stretching exercise shown here will help relieve stress if practiced on a regular basis. It stretches the chest muscles, allowing the lungs to fill with more oxygen and relieving stress-induced pressure across the chest.

1 *Stand with your feet together and arms by your sides.*

2 *Take a deep breath and raise your arms slowly.*

3 *Rise up onto your toes as you raise your arms to meet above your head. Repeat twice.*

PHYSICAL BENEFITS OF EXERCISE

Regular exercise provides many physical benefits that help the body to work more efficiently and reduce the risk of developing a number of life-threatening diseases.

The major health benefits of physical activity were spelled out in a 1995 report from the Department of Health and Human Services in the United States. Regular exercise not only reduces the risk of some disorders, including heart disease, high blood pressure, diabetes, and cancer of the colon, but also increases life expectancy and the possibility of fulfilling it healthfully

Exercise improves posture, strengthens the back, and helps to maintain healthy bones, muscles, and joints, reducing the risk of arthritis and helping older adults become stronger and better able to move about safely and independently. It also helps speed the recovery process following childbirth and various illnesses, builds up energy levels, and helps to control weight.

THE CARDIOVASCULAR SYSTEM

The most basic measure of health and fitness is the efficiency of the cardiovascular system, the network of blood vessels with the heart at its center. The heart pumps blood through the arteries, circulating oxygen throughout the body and bringing it back through the veins. During exercise the muscles demand more oxygen, which forces the heart to work harder and pump more blood around the body. Over time this improves the heart's strength and efficiency. Regular training helps the heart to beat more strongly, which in turn allows it to beat more slowly. A slow heartbeat is a sign that a heart is healthy, because it doesn't have to work so hard to circulate the blood.

Comparing the heart rate of a sedentary person with that of a physically trained one shows some major differences. At rest, the average adult must have about 5 liters (5 quarts) of blood per minute pumped around the body. In a sedentary person this could demand a heart rate of 80 or more beats per minute, and the stroke volume (amount of blood ejected from the heart per beat) would be about 70 milliliters (2½ fluid ounces) or less. By contrast, in a physically

HOW YOUR HEART WORKS

Your heart is divided into four chambers—the two atria and the two ventricles—and acts as a pump. The two chambers on the right side of the heart receive blood from the body's tissues after it is depleted of oxygen and pump it to the lungs, where the oxygen is replaced. The chambers on the left side of the heart receive the oxygen-rich blood from the lungs and then pump it back around the body.

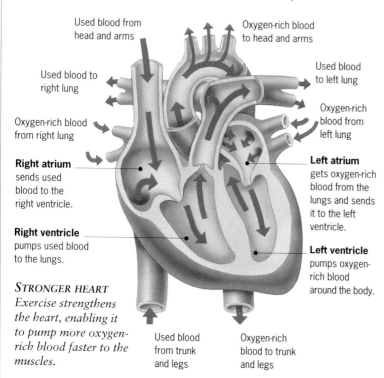

Used blood from head and arms

Oxygen-rich blood to head and arms

Used blood to right lung

Used blood to left lung

Oxygen-rich blood from right lung

Oxygen-rich blood from left lung

Right atrium sends used blood to the right ventricle.

Left atrium gets oxygen-rich blood from the lungs and sends it to the left ventricle.

Right ventricle pumps used blood to the lungs.

Left ventricle pumps oxygen-rich blood around the body.

STRONGER HEART Exercise strengthens the heart, enabling it to pump more oxygen-rich blood faster to the muscles.

Used blood from trunk and legs

Oxygen-rich blood to trunk and legs

ASTHMA AND EXERCISE

Many people who suffer from asthma think that exercise in any form will only exacerbate their condition. This, however, is untrue. Although breathlessness and wheezing cannot be eradicated through exercise alone, the deep-breathing techniques and controlled regular breaths required by exercise such as yoga or swimming can help to improve lung function. These exercises also ease tense muscles, widen the airways, and promote overall relaxation, which in turn can lower stress levels and help reduce the number and severity of asthma attacks.

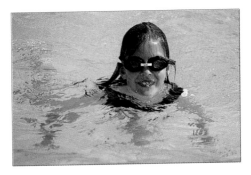

TAKE THE PLUNGE
Swimming is an excellent exercise for the muscles that also strengthens the respiratory system and fosters controlled breathing.

Boost your lungs
Many people quickly run out of breath when they exert themselves. Exercise can improve the elasticity of the lungs and thus make better and more efficient use of the respiratory system.

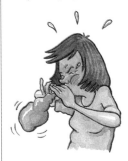

SHALLOW BREATHING
During normal breathing the lungs move just 500 milliliters (about a pint) of air with each breath.

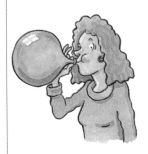

DEEP BREATHS
During strenuous exercise lung capacity increases to 2½ to 3½ liters (about 2½ to 3½ quarts).

fit person the stroke volume would be much greater—100 to 200 milliliters (3½ to 7 fluid ounces)—and the heart rate much lower at 40 to 50 beats per minute. This means that the heart is pumping out more blood with each beat and working less hard to deliver the blood the body needs.

Top long-distance runners have a greatly enlarged heart size and can achieve a cardiac output as high as 40 liters (about 40 quarts) per minute. They may have a resting heart rate of 30 beats per minute or even less.

THE RESPIRATORY SYSTEM

Exercise can improve the efficiency of the respiratory system by increasing lung capacity. Under normal conditions only a small part—about one-quarter—of total lung capacity is used (see far right).

Training, especially during adolescence, when the lungs are still developing, can significantly increase their dimensions and improve their capacity for delivering oxygen to the blood. These improvements can then be maintained throughout adult life, even after training has ceased. Activities that require the development of enhanced breathing capacity lead to the greatest increases in lung volume; divers and people who learned to play a wind instrument when young usually have the largest lungs.

Available lung volume usually begins to decline after age 30, owing to the loss of tissue elasticity. However, most tissues respond to the demands placed upon them, and the lungs are no exception. The age-related decline in lung function can be slowed by exercise.

THE LYMPHATIC SYSTEM

The lymphatic system is the cornerstone of your immunity. It is a barrier to the spread of infection and harmful bacteria—the more efficiently it works, the healthier you are. The system is a series of connected vessels containing lymph fluid, a watery substance that bathes all the tissues of the body. This fluid contains the white cells that help to combat infection, along with any harmful microorganisms that might be present.

Unlike blood, which is pumped by the heart muscle, lymph relies solely on physical movement for its circulation. Any activity, therefore, improves lymph activity. For example, the repeated waves of gravitational pull exerted on your body when bouncing on a trampoline act like a pump and promote better lymphatic functioning.

THE BRAIN

Doctors and scientists have long noted changes to the cardiovascular and muscular systems brought about by exercise. More recently, however, there has been a growing realization that changes in psychological function also accompany regular exercise. The study of these adaptations is still in its infancy, partly due to the practical difficulties of measuring the changes, but also because our understanding of normal brain function is still relatively poor.

What is clear, however, is that most persons who engage in regular exercise report an improved sense of well-being. This probably has a chemical basis, and there is now some evidence to suggest that exercise produces changes in the sensitivity of some of

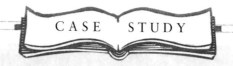

Returning to Exercise

As many people age, they find that they steadily gain weight. Generally, this happens not because they are eating more than before but because their lifestyle has become more sedentary without a corresponding reduction in food intake. The best way to tackle such weight gain is to take up exercise again, but this requires preparation and a gradual buildup.

Joe is 48 and married with three children; his eldest, Paul, is married and has seven-year-old twins. Joe was a keen soccer player in his younger days, but he hasn't played for 20 years and now does little exercise. Recently his job as a sales manager has become more demanding. Because he spends long hours at the office, he often misses the evening meal at home and snacks on chips, takeout food, and sweets instead.

Although he won't admit it, he's becoming extremely conscious of his expanding waistline. As a starting point to improving his health, he decided to play a game of soccer with his grandchildren one weekend and was horrified to find himself breathless after only a few minutes.

WHAT SHOULD JOE DO?

Joe went to see his doctor, who told him that he was overweight, that his blood pressure was a little on the high side, and his cholesterol level was elevated. However, the doctor found no medical reason why Joe should not embark on an exercise program. He advised him to start gradually, with a less strenuous form of exercise than soccer. He also told Joe to improve his diet and try to lose weight by cutting back on high-fat food and sweets and eating more fruits, vegetables, and complex carbohydrates, preferably whole grain.

The doctor recommended that Joe start a regimen of gentle walking for the first few weeks, gradually building up in intensity to a slow jog within a month.

HEALTH
Lack of exercise can aggravate many health problems, such as high cholesterol and high blood pressure.

DIET
The wrong type of food combined with a sedentary lifestyle is a recipe for ill health and a lack of general fitness.

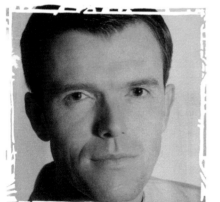

FITNESS
Undertaking strenuous exercise after a long break can bring on unpleasant physical symptoms.

Action Plan

HEALTH
Have regular checkups to monitor cholesterol and blood pressure levels.

DIET
Cut down on high-fat foods and sweets and eat more vegetables, fruits, and starches, especially whole-grain ones like brown rice and whole-wheat bread.

FITNESS
Start a fitness program, initially doing gentle exercise. Gradually build up the intensity and time until fit enough to carry out more strenuous forms of exercise.

HOW THINGS TURNED OUT FOR JOE

Joe started to take a 30-minute walk every lunchtime, which helped with both his weight and his breathlessness. His new diet improved his energy levels, and after three months a medical checkup revealed a slight improvement in his cholesterol levels and blood pressure. A recent game of soccer with his grandchildren left him pleasantly tired and relaxed rather than breathless, and he is considering joining a soccer team for older players.

MUSCLE CHANGES THROUGH USE AND DISUSE

Muscle is one of the most elastic of all the body's tissues. Designed to expand to cope with increased physical activity, it rapidly adapts to exercise. Changes in the structure and function of muscle are apparent after as little as one week of a training program involving a gradually increasing exercise load.

Contrary to popular belief, unused muscles do not turn to fat, but any muscle that is not used will atrophy, or decrease in size, as muscle fibers waste away. Reduced activity means less energy expenditure, but unfortunately, the appetite does not shrink accordingly, and if food intake continues at the previous level, an increase in body fat will occur alongside the loss of muscle mass. The good news is that these changes are easily reversed by a return to the previous level of activity.

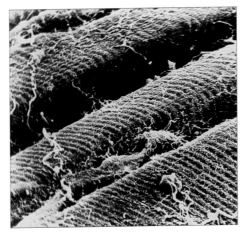

Skeletal Muscle
Muscle that is responsible for physical action is known as skeletal, or striated (striped), muscle, shown above. Skeletal muscle is in a constant state of tension, called muscle tone, and needs to be kept active or it will shrink and start to be covered by a layer of fat.

the brain cells to neurotransmitter agents (the chemical messengers that enable brain cells to communicate with each other). These changes may have implications for enhancing mood and coping with stress.

THE MUSCLES

Some of the characteristics of your muscles are determined by genetic makeup, but major changes can be produced by training. The response of muscles to exercise depends on the form of training undertaken; it can increase muscle size, strength, or endurance or a combination of these. A bodybuilder's training program results in large, well-defined muscles; training for weight lifting does not lead to such size increases but produces strong muscles that are capable of generating greater force. A marathon runner's training does not increase muscle size either but results in muscles that can be kept active for long periods without tiring.

Training regimens for the average person are designed to improve health and well-being by increasing both strength and endurance, but they tend to focus on the cardiovascular benefits that accompany aerobic training (see page 35). Strength training should not be neglected, however. Muscular strength can be significantly improved without a large increase in muscle size. Muscle strength usually declines with age, but this is largely a result of the reduced activity that normally occurs as we get older. Remaining active will preserve muscle strength, helping you to keep your independence into old age.

BONES

After young adulthood there is a progressive loss of calcium from the bones, which results in a diminishing of bone strength. This occurrence affects both women and men but is a more serious concern for women. There are two reasons for this. First, women live longer than men on average and so are more likely to live to an age at which the loss of bone mineral becomes serious. Second, the hormone estrogen plays an important role in maintaining bone density in women. After menopause the level of estrogen in the blood diminishes, leading to a higher rate of calcium loss and increased demineralization.

An adequate intake of calcium and vitamin D in the diet is essential for providing the raw minerals for building bones, but regular exercise is also important because it ensures that these minerals are converted into bone. When a bone is put under stress during exercise, it responds by becoming thicker and stronger; that is, it increases its mass. Exercise during the early years of life

A STRONGER, LEANER LOOK WITH TRAINING
The 1970s tennis star Chris Evert illustrated the dramatic changes possible in muscle tone and strength through a combination of aerobic and anaerobic training. She developed a leaner and more defined physical appearance by changing her training to build up muscle and reduce excess body fat.

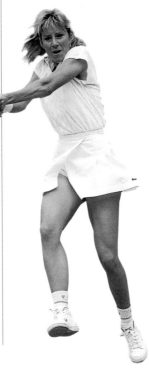

is particularly important because it increases the peak bone mass, which is normally reached between the ages of 20 and 30.

Continuing exercise after this point will slow the rate of bone loss. The most effective types of exercise are those that place stress on the bones, such as jogging and aerobics. If you are just starting out on an exercise program, however, begin these activities at a moderate level and increase slowly so that the bones, muscles, and joints have time to adjust.

METABOLIC ADAPTATIONS TO EXERCISE

Regular exercise has a direct effect on your body's metabolic rate—that is, the amount of energy your body uses to fuel all bodily functions. Your metabolic rate rises during exercise and gradually falls afterward. There is evidence to suggest that it remains above the resting level for between 12 and 24 hours if exercise is prolonged and performed close to the maximum intensity that can be sustained. These results apply more to distance runners, cyclists, or swimmers engaged in hard training than to recreational exercisers. However, the cumulative effect of even small elevations in the metabolic rate seems to be important over the long term and can contribute to weight loss.

Weight loss and weight control

One of the biggest metabolic changes that occurs with regular aerobic exercise is a switch in the fuel mixture that the body uses to power the muscles during exercise. Muscles are normally fueled by a mixture of fat and carbohydrates, which is broken down in the presence of oxygen to produce carbon dioxide and water. The energy released during combustion is then available for the muscles to use.

At moderate exercise intensities, only a small contribution comes from carbohydrates, whereas fat is the major fuel. Some of the fat used comes from the small stores within working muscles, but most comes via the blood from the large stores contained in the adipose tissue beneath the skin and around internal organs like the kidneys. As the intensity of exercise increases, however, there is a gradual increase in the proportion of energy that carbohydrates supply and a decreased contribution from fat. This is good news if you are overweight because it

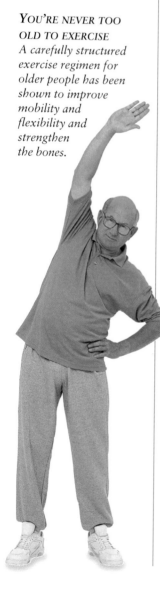

YOU'RE NEVER TOO OLD TO EXERCISE
A carefully structured exercise regimen for older people has been shown to improve mobility and flexibility and strengthen the bones.

Origins

A team at the Medical Research Council in the United Kingdom, led by Professor Jerry Morris, was the first to prove a link between inactivity and the risk of heart attack. In a long-term study into the lifestyle of thousands of civil servants, they found that those engaged in active leisure pursuits, such as brisk walking, swimming, or badminton, even if only on the weekend, had one-third the risk of heart attack as those who led completely sedentary lives.

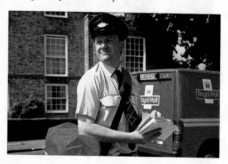

ROUTE TO GOOD HEALTH
A link between exercise and health was first discovered during research into jobs conducted in the late 1940s. Mail carriers, for example, were found to be at less risk for heart disease than office workers.

means that you need not feel pressured into performing high-intensity exercise; activity of moderate intensity, such as brisk walking or cycling, is a good way to lose fat.

EXERCISE AND AGING

Exercise not only helps prevent or relieve age-related illnesses, such as osteoporosis and arthritis, but also leads to greater independence in old age. A 1994 study of residents in a nursing home with an average age of 98 years showed that they could improve their fitness with a graded weight training program. Using elastic training straps that provide gentle resistance, they were able to increase their muscular strength significantly. Not only did this improve their independence, allowing them to do things for themselves that had previously been impossible—such as getting up from a chair unaided—but the improved strength was accompanied by a better sense of balance and a reduced risk of falling.

PSYCHOLOGICAL BENEFITS OF EXERCISE

Regular exercise provides clear psychological benefits, including improvements in self-confidence and mental alertness and the alleviation of mood disorders such as anxiety and depression.

The psychological benefits of exercise can be just as valid and important as the physical ones; for some people they may even become the most rewarding aspect of their training. Exercise produces these beneficial effects in two general ways: it counteracts the negative effects of excess stress, and it acts as a mood enhancer, often creating an emotional high for the exerciser.

STRESS REDUCTION

A certain degree of stress is inevitable and even desirable because it can act as a spur toward greater achievement and improve physical performance by accelerating the body's metabolism. However, excess levels of stress can have a negative impact on the body and even cause something as major as a heart attack. Exercise can play an important role in reducing these negative effects.

Your body's stress response is designed to help you deal with physical danger. In a stressful situation adrenaline and noradrenaline are released, providing you with extra energy; your heart rate speeds up and your blood pressure rises, your liver releases glucose for energy, and all senses are sharpened as your body experiences a state of extra alertness. All these physiological changes require a physical release; if stress is allowed to build up, physical damage and unpleasant mental tension can follow.

Continuous high levels of stress hormones in the blood make your heart work harder and keep your blood pressure elevated. In the long term these same hormones raise blood fat and cholesterol levels and cause arteries to become clogged with fatty deposits, increasing the risk of a heart attack or stroke. Long-term stress can weaken the immune system as well, making you more prone to infection, and it can lead to depression because unrelieved tension and anxiety, combined with fatigue, affect the balance of chemicals in the brain. The physiological stress reaction is ideal for exercise, however, because it prepares your body for extreme exertion, and a challenging game of tennis or even a very brisk walk will utilize your body's additional energy reserves. The effectiveness of exercise in

---

STRESS THROUGHOUT HISTORY

The stress response is partly a throwback to earlier, more primitive times. It is designed to ensure that your body is at its peak of physical efficiency and thus increase your chances of survival when threatened. In the days of our ancient ancestors, problems that triggered the stress response, like an attack by wild animals or marauding tribes, could be resolved only by violent action or rapid escape—in other words, fight or flight. But the causes of stress today are more likely to involve mental pressures, such as too much work or financial worries, and to require a nonphysical solution. Exercise provides a vital release valve to prevent a harmful buildup of unresolved physical tension.

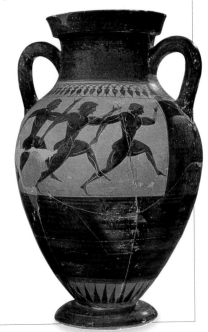

FIGHT OR FLIGHT
The ancient Greeks recognized that people under stress can achieve amazing feats in sports or battles; many Greek vase paintings celebrate the prowess of athletes and warriors. The stress factor still plays a part in competition today, demonstrated by athletes who break records during major events.

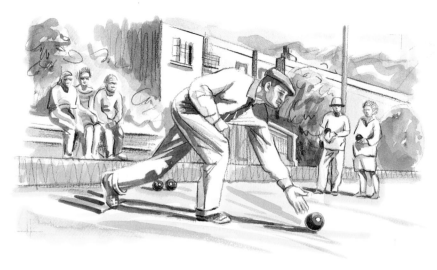

STRESS RELIEF
Sports do not have to be strenuous to improve mood and relieve stress. Activities like lawn bowling provide many beneficial emotional effects, both through the physical effort involved and the social opportunities that they afford.

helping to control physical responses to stress has been measured in athletes and other persons who are physically fit. The results show that people who exercise regularly have lower pulse rates under stressful conditions than those who are less fit.

IMPROVED MOOD

As tension and anxiety are released, a state of relaxation follows, leading to a positive sense of well-being and euphoria. Explanations for this lift in mood vary. One is that simply relieving stress is responsible for much of the improvement in mood that most people report after exercising. Various changes take place—breathing deepens, replacing the typically shallow and fast breathing that accompanies stress; levels of norepinephrine, an emotion stabilizer, increase; and muscles relax through the release of tension-causing hormones.

Another widely accepted explanation is the theory of the "runner's high." This is based on the fact that prolonged exercise releases mood-enhancing chemicals called endorphins, which in turn induce a state of euphoria (see right).

Yet another notion, the thermogenic theory, attributes lower levels of tension to an increase in body temperature, which in turn affects brain waves.

The neurotransmitter theory suggests that exercise increases the sensitivity of serotonin receptors in the brain, making these naturally produced chemical messengers more effective at reducing pain. An experiment on mood and exercise conducted in 1993 showed that after exercise, brain serotonin increased and was followed by a reduction in appetite and relief from depression.

In addition to its effect on a person's emotional state, regular exercise promotes a rise in self-esteem through an increasingly improved body image and greater self-confidence. As you gain a sense of self-empowerment in completing an exercise and improving a physical skill—and at the same time are diverted from other daily concerns and stresses—you will become more emotionally stable and self-sufficient.

SOCIAL OPPORTUNITIES

There is a long-standing impression that the devoted athlete is a solitary individual, but exercise can be beneficial as a means of social interaction. Although there are undoubtedly some people who prefer to exercise alone, exercise in general offers many social opportunities, both during the activity itself and afterward.

Whatever your favored choice of sport or exercise, there is probably a club associated with it where participants can meet. The shared goals and sense of achievement of fellow sports people create powerful bonds, and membership in a club also brings the realization that there are many others with ambitions similar to your own. Joining a club often makes an important contribution in the early stages of an exercise program, when the encouragement of others who have been through the same experiences can be of great help and can save a beginner from many mistakes.

EXERCISE AND ENDORPHINS

Many people who exercise regularly report that they often achieve a feeling of euphoria, or a meditative, trance-like state of altered consciousness. There is still much that is not clearly understood about this effect, which is often referred to as a "runner's high," but it has been linked to the release of endorphins—the body's natural painkilling chemicals.

Although this idea still remains controversial, a number of studies indicate that 30 to 60 minutes of constant moderate to intense exercise does indeed increase endorphin levels, which in turn reduce anxiety, sensitivity to pain, depression, and stress.

A Grieving Widower

Encountering any of life's major stresses, such as losing a loved one or moving to a new house, can have a profound effect not only on mental health but also on physical well-being. Rather than turn to conventional medicine and drugs as an antidote to stress, depression, or anguish, many people choose exercise, which offers a more attractive alternative.

Ted is a 64-year-old former teacher who took early retirement because he was feeling unable to cope with another term in the classroom. He was looking forward to a long retirement with his wife, Sue, and was devastated when she developed breast cancer and died less than a year later. The trauma of loss was gradually replaced by an acute sense of loneliness, accompanied by growing isolation and depression. Because Ted and Sue had been content with each other's company, they had never felt the need for many friends. Also, Sue was a keen cook, but Ted now eats ready-made meals from the supermarket. After three years on his own, Ted began to experience recurring chest pains and went to see his doctor.

WHAT SHOULD TED DO?

After a thorough physical exam, Ted's doctor pronounced him to be in reasonably good physical shape. His electrocardiogram was fine, and his blood cholesterol levels were normal. His blood pressure was slightly above the recommended range, but he was not overweight. It was only while discussing these results with Ted that the doctor realized Ted's physical symptoms were probably a manifestation of his unhappiness.

Ted expected his doctor to prescribe medication and was going to resist this suggestion. He was very surprised when instead the doctor told him that he just needed to get some exercise. He gave Ted the name of a fitness instructor at the local senior center to contact.

Action Plan

EXERCISE
Take up some form of social exercise or fitness program that involves contact and interaction with other people.

DIET
Start browsing through cookbooks and take a class to learn how to prepare food. Have people over to share a meal.

STRESS
Focus your attention on physical exercise and interaction with other people to turn your mind away from continually thinking about how lonely you are.

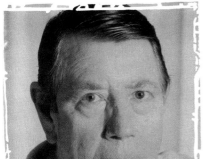

STRESS
Emotional turmoil and tension can increase heart rate and blood pressure. Worrying about these conditions simply adds to the burden.

DIET
A monotonous and poor diet will deplete the body of vitamins and minerals needed to maintain your emotional and physical health.

EXERCISE
Lack of regular exercise can block the release of pent-up emotions and intensify stress levels.

HOW THINGS TURNED OUT FOR TED

Ted joined an aerobics class for seniors, which he attended twice a week. As he became fitter and began to exercise more, his chest pains disappeared and he started to take more interest in his meals. He made a point of selecting healthy, low-fat options and also learned some cooking skills. He was able to put these to good use during social evenings at the senior center, for which members took turns preparing the meals.

PREVENTING DISEASE WITH EXERCISE

Regular exercise not only provides many general health benefits but also helps prevent or relieve a number of specific illnesses and diseases.

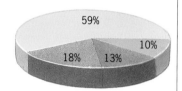

RISK FACTORS FOR HEART DISEASE
According to a U.S. survey, inactivity is the most significant factor in the development of heart disease, affecting 59 percent of the population. The next most harmful factor is smoking (18 percent), followed by high cholesterol (10 percent); all other factors grouped together total 13 percent.

Much recent research has focused on the major contribution that regular exercise can make to preventing or limiting the severity of several serious conditions and disorders. These include heart disease, elevated cholesterol, high blood pressure, and diabetes mellitus.

CORONARY HEART DISEASE
The major cause of death in most of the industrialized countries, heart disease accounts for half again as many deaths as cancer, which is the second most common cause. Even in young adults, heart disease is a major killer. American statistics show that in the age range of 25 to 44, only accidents rank higher as a cause of death. In Canada heart disease and stroke claim more than 79,000 lives annually. Death rates from heart disease are largely related to lifestyle factors, including diet, smoking, stress, and habitual low levels of exercise. Although much emphasis is placed on the first three, the evidence now available shows that physical inactivity may in fact be the most significant factor contributing to heart disease.

There is compelling evidence that regular physical activity, even in modest amounts, can help lower blood pressure and cholesterol and contribute to a decreased risk of dying prematurely from a heart attack. People who exercise regularly also have a reduced tendency to form blood clots, which can precipitate a heart attack or stroke.

HIGH BLOOD CHOLESTEROL
A high blood cholesterol level has been linked with an increased likelihood of suffering a heart attack. The main risk comes from excess levels of a substance called low-density lipoprotein (LDL), which deposits cholesterol in the arteries and clogs them. Another substance, high-density lipoprotein (HDL), is more beneficial because it tends to prevent the buildup of cholesterol in the arteries. It is important for good health, therefore, to have low overall cholesterol levels in the blood and, in particular, a blood profile that is low in LDL and relatively high in HDL.

Evidence suggests that exercise reduces overall cholesterol levels and produces a favorable shift in the blood profile from LDLs to HDLs. The complete picture, however, is a bit more complicated because there is also a link between the degree of body fat and blood cholesterol levels. Those who exercise on a regular basis tend to be leaner than average, and thus the finding of low LDL and high HDL levels is to be

BLOOD PRESSURE AND EXERCISE

Blood pressure readings show the elasticity of the arteries, which can harden and narrow as a result of age and disease. Abnormally high blood pressure indicates an increased risk of heart disease, stroke, and kidney disease. Exercise helps to keep arteries healthier and more elastic, resulting in lower blood pressure and a reduced risk of illness.

MEASURING BLOOD PRESSURE
Blood pressure monitoring involves two readings registered in millimeters of mercury, or mm Hg—systolic, or maximum, pressure and diastolic, or minimum, pressure. An unfit person may have a reading of 170/105 mm Hg or higher, while a person who exercises regulary may have a lower reading, like 120/85 mm Hg.

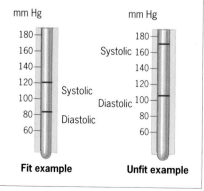

Fit example   **Unfit example**

CHOLESTEROL AND EXERCISE

A substance in the blood called low-density lipoprotein (LDL) is partly responsible for depositing fatty plaques on artery walls, causing them to narrow and restrict blood flow, which can lead to a heart attack or stroke. High-density lipoprotein (HDL), however, helps carry cholesterol away from the artery walls to the liver, where it is turned into bile and used in digestion or removed from the body.

BLOOD CHOLESTEROL
Exercise encourages a shift from the development of "bad" LDL to "good" HDL in the body.

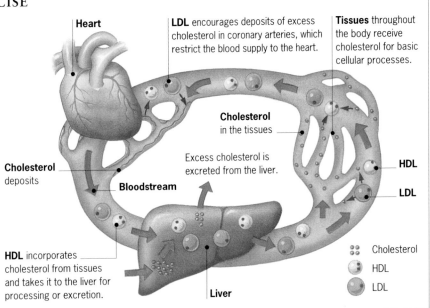

Heart

LDL encourages deposits of excess cholesterol in coronary arteries, which restrict the blood supply to the heart.

Tissues throughout the body receive cholesterol for basic cellular processes.

Cholesterol in the tissues

Excess cholesterol is excreted from the liver.

Cholesterol deposits

Bloodstream

HDL

LDL

HDL incorporates cholesterol from tissues and takes it to the liver for processing or excretion.

Liver

Cholesterol
HDL
LDL

---

expected. However, even after differences in body fat are accounted for, the evidence still indicates that those who exercise have a more favorable blood cholesterol profile.

OBESITY

There is overwhelming evidence that obesity is a contributing cause to a number of common disorders, including heart disease and type II, or adult-onset, diabetes. Statistics show that obese people are twice as likely to die of heart disease as their slimmer counterparts. In addition, many overweight people are dissatisfied with their condition, and in some cases this can lead to psychological and emotional problems.

The usual approach to losing weight is to reduce calorie intake, but the weight loss that results is generally small and in many cases proves to be temporary. Severe dieting is often accompanied by feelings of weakness and tiredness that discourage physical activity, but without exercise the body will lose muscle tissue during periods of restricted energy intake. This loss of muscle leads to a lowered metabolic rate, which further reduces energy requirements, making it even more difficult to lose weight.

A better approach to weight control is to increase energy expenditure through exercise while restricting the types of food eaten. A diet that is low in fat and high in protein and whole-grain complex carbohydrates, together with regular exercise, will maintain

muscle while reducing weight. The best approach is to choose a form of exercise that is within your capabilities and does not place undue stress on the joints—swimming and walking, for example, are ideal. The energy consumed by walking is proportional to body weight, so even walking a short distance is effective when your body weight is high. Your capacity will be limited at first, but increasing levels of fitness will allow you eventually to perform more exercise without discomfort.

DIABETES MELLITUS

Diabetes mellitus is the result of a failure of the body to produce or use the hormone insulin in sufficient amounts to regulate the supply of glucose to the tissues. This leads to large swings in blood sugar levels. There are two main forms of diabetes. Type I, or insulin-dependent, diabetes usually develops in young people and is controlled by regular insulin injections. Type II, or noninsulin-dependent, diabetes develops mainly in adults over 40 and may require oral medication to control it.

With suitable attention to diet and perhaps some alteration to the medication regimen, diabetic individuals can usually take part in sports and exercise. Indeed, a number of top sports figures are diabetic. Many diabetics who exercise regularly report better control of their blood sugar levels and a
continued on page 30

LOSING WEIGHT
Cycling is a good form of exercise for overweight people; it is aerobic, so it helps burn calories, but it is nonimpact, so it puts minimal strain on joints.

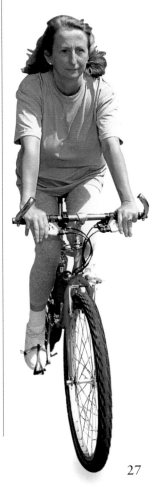

Diabetes Mellitus

Diabetes mellitus results from a problem with insulin, the hormone that enables tissues to utilize glucose for energy. There is no cure, but a healthy diet and regular exercise can help diabetics to manage the condition and lead healthy, active lives.

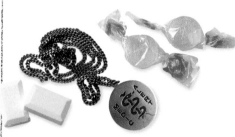

ESSENTIAL EQUIPMENT
An identification bracelet, medication, and emergency carbohydrates are essential items for diabetics to carry.

DIABETES AND TOP-CLASS PLAYERS

Soccer player Gary Mabbutt has had insulin-dependent diabetes since he was 17. He has to monitor his blood sugar levels regularly, inject himself with insulin four times a day, and follow a carefully controlled diet. Nevertheless, diabetes has not hindered his training nor success, and he has had a long career in top-level soccer, having captained Tottenham Hotspur for more than 10 years and played 16 games for England.

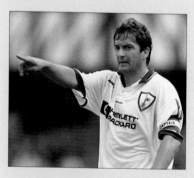

GARY MABBUTT
Diabetic athletes like Gary Mabbutt must check their blood glucose before and after a game and at halftime and, if necessary, eat a snack to keep sugar levels steady.

Exercise is of great benefit to all diabetics, who often have high blood pressure and high cholesterol in addition to their disease and are at increased risk for heart disease. Many are also overweight. Regular moderate exercise can aid in control of blood sugar, lower blood pressure and cholesterol levels, assist weight loss, and reduce the risk of heart disease. For some sufferers exercise can even help restore blood glucose to normal or near normal levels.

There are two main types of diabetes, each requiring different forms of treatment. Most sufferers of Type II, or noninsulin-dependent, diabetes manage the condition with diet and hypoglycemic tablets or diet alone. However, the 10 percent who have Type I, or insulin-dependent, diabetes must have daily insulin injections as well as a controlled diet.

Whichever type of diabetes you have, you must seek the advice of your doctor before starting an exercise program because exercise will rapidly lower blood glucose levels and possibly cause hypoglycemia, or low blood sugar. Symptoms of hypoglycemia include shaking, sweating, blurred or double vision, and slurred speech. In this situation extra sugar in the form of glucose tablets, sugar lumps, chocolate, or sweet tea will relieve the symptoms. In severe cases the sufferer may lose consciousness and require emergency treatment.

If you are taking hypoglycemic tablets, you should also consult a doctor about exercise. While you are not at as much risk of hypoglycemia as insulin-dependent diabetics, exercise can still take your blood glucose to dangerously low levels.

A SENSIBLE EATING PLAN FOR DIABETICS

Diabetics need individual advice from a dietitian, but the principles of eating are similar to the guidelines advised for everyone. Starchy foods like bread, rice, and pasta should make up the bulk of a meal plan but be eaten in small quantities at regular intervals to avoid dramatic swings in glucose levels. Your nutritionist will advise you on the amounts that are safe for you to consume at each meal and have you follow the glycemic index (see page 46), which rates carbohydrates according to the speed with which each one breaks down. A food with a high number, such as a potato, banana, or white rice, should be balanced with one that has a lower number, like a dairy product or beans. Including plenty of high-fiber foods is also important.

Foods and drinks containing refined sugar, which cause a rapid rise in blood glucose levels, should be avoided except in an emergency to counteract a dangerous drop in blood glucose. Sweets containing artificial sweeteners are acceptable.

Eating regular meals helps prevent wide swings in blood glucose. Many diabetics also need snacks midmorning, midafternoon, and at bedtime.

EXERCISE FOR DIABETICS

Before beginning any exercise program, it's advisable to discuss your plans with your doctor and have an exercise treadmill test. Your diet may have to be adjusted to make sure that it contains enough energy for the level of activity you plan. Also, if your blood pressure is even slightly elevated, it can rise higher with exercise; to start, you should work out at no more than 50 to 65 percent of your maximum heart rate.

If you are unused to exercise, choose an aerobic activity that you can easily incorporate into your lifestyle. Start with 5 minutes a day, and as your fitness improves, gradually extend the sessions to 20 to 30 minutes three to five days a week.

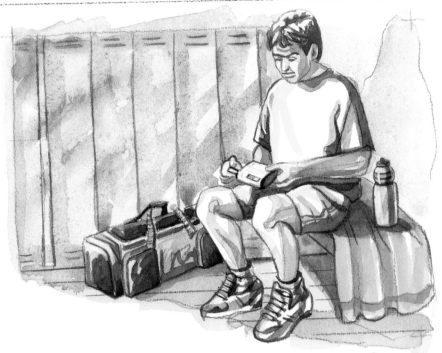

Diabetes treated with tablets

Hypoglycemic tablets and exercise both reduce blood glucose, so levels can drop too low. Try to exercise when blood glucose levels are at their highest—usually an hour after a meal—and have your next scheduled meal or snack shortly after strenuous exercise. Monitor your blood glucose before and after exercise. If the levels are persistently low, your doctor may have to reduce your dosage. Carry diabetic identification and emergency carbohydrates with you at all times.

Diabetes treated with insulin

Exercise quickly lowers glucose levels in insulin-dependent diabetics, so you may be advised to eat extra carbohydrates before and during workouts. What and how much depends on the type and duration of the activity. Short bursts of activity may require a rapid source of energy, such as a chocolate bar, sugar candy, or glucose tablets. For more prolonged exercise you may need a starchy carbohydrate, like a peanut butter sandwich. Extra carbohydrates may also be needed after exercise.

Monitor your blood glucose before and after exercising and, if necessary, during the session as well. Regular exercise may require a reduction in your insulin dosage. Inject insulin about an hour before exercise but not into a muscle that will be exerted because this may alter its effect.

Always carry diabetic identification and a carbohydrate, such as glucose tablets, and make sure that people close to you know what to do in an emergency. Many diabetics carry glucagon with them. This prescription hormone boosts sugar levels and can rouse an unconscious diabetic.

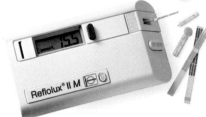

BLOOD GLUCOSE MONITORING
Electronic devices are available that make it easier for diabetics to monitor their blood glucose levels before, after, and even during an exercise session.

ESSENTIAL FOOT CARE

Everyone should follow good hygiene practices in the locker room, but it is especially vital for diabetics to do so. Poor foot care in particular can lead to serious complications because diabetics are prone to foot infections, foot ulcers, and in extreme cases, gangrene (tissue death). To prevent infection, follow scrupulous daily hygiene, wear sandals in the shower, and never walk barefoot. Do not cut corns or calluses, and to avoid blisters, wear cushioned socks and comfortable shoes. Seek immediate treatment if a foot infection develops.

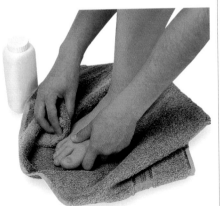

PREVENTING FOOT INFECTIONS
Always dry the feet carefully and use foot creams and powders to keep the skin supple and prevent cracking.

Exercise for relieving symptoms of PMS

Regular exercise can reduce the symptoms of premenstrual syndrome (PMS), including fatigue, headache, and general discomfort. The main reason for this effect is that exercise helps prevent fluid retention by relocating any excess fluid from tissues back into the bloodstream.

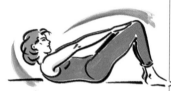

PELVIC TILTS
Lie on the floor with knees bent and about hip width apart. Breathe out, tucking your chin in, and push your lower back against the floor while raising your pubic bone. Repeat 10 times.

ABDOMINAL CURLS
Start as for the pelvic tilt but rest your hands on your thighs. As you breathe out and perform a pelvic tilt, curl your head and shoulders off the floor, sliding your hands up your thighs. Count to four, then slide back down slowly. Repeat 10 times.

reduction in the amount of insulin needed. The tissues of athletes are more sensitive to the effects of insulin than those of untrained persons, so they need less insulin to regulate the responses of the body to ingested food. Provided that sensible precautions are taken and that the program builds up gradually, every individual diagnosed as diabetic should be encouraged to become more active.

LUNG DISORDERS

People with lung disorders, such as chronic bronchitis, emphysema, or asthma, have limited tolerance for exercise. Nevertheless, exercise can bring about major physical and psychological benefits.

Exercise tolerance can be increased with medication, through conscious control of the breathing pattern, and by the increase in muscular strength and endurance that occurs with the exercise itself. A regimen of regular aerobic exercise is particularly beneficial because it increases the general level of fitness, thus reducing the need for strenuous breathing at lower levels of exertion.

OSTEOPOROSIS

The incidence of osteoporosis among older women is becoming much more widespread. Fractures, particularly of the hip or wrist as a consequence of falls, are a major cause of hospitalization and can lead to further complications. There is normally a progressive loss of bone in later life. If this continues

over a prolonged period, the bone may eventually deteriorate to the point where fractures occur easily.

Exercise cannot completely prevent the gradual loss of bone in later life, but vigorous exercise during childhood and up to about 35 years of age ensures the buildup of a high peak bone mass, so the bone has further to deteriorate before it becomes brittle. In addition, a sensible exercise program from the late thirties onward will slow the rate of demineralization.

OTHER BENEFITS

Exercise improves blood circulation to the brain, thus improving brain function. This is particularly important in the elderly because there is evidence that regular exercise may slow the decline in mental performance that can accompany old age.

Patients with kidney disease have reported improvement in kidney function after beginning exercise, and their mental attitude has also improved.

There is convincing evidence of a reduced risk of developing colon cancer among people who exercise regularly, and some surveys have shown a direct relationship between physical fitness levels and death rates from all types of cancer. The major benefit may be a secondary one, in that regular exercise may help promote lifestyle changes, like quitting smoking, which lead in turn to a reduced risk of cancer.

EXERCISES FOR PREVENTING OSTEOPOROSIS

Regular exercise helps to maintain bone density. Many of the stresses imposed on bones during exercise strengthen them and make them more resistant to weakening. The spine-strengthening exercises shown below will help to reduce the potential for osteoporosis-related curvature of the spine.

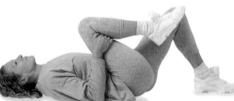

1 *Lying on your back, bring both knees as close as possible to your chest, hold for 5 seconds, then lower your legs back down. Working with only one leg at a time, repeat the stretch 10 times.*

2 *Lying on your back with your knees bent, raise your head and shoulders off the floor, push the small of your back as hard as you can against the floor, and hold for 5 seconds. Repeat 10 times.*

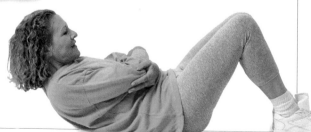

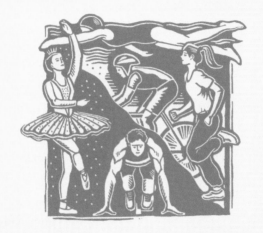

CHAPTER 2

EXERCISE FACTS

You do not need a comprehensive knowledge of the physiology of exercise in order to become fit, but an understanding of the basics, such as the components of fitness and the difference between aerobic and anaerobic exercise, will allow you to tailor your fitness program specifically to your personal needs.

DIFFERENT TYPES OF EXERCISE

There are two main types of exercise—anaerobic and aerobic. Because they utilize different energy systems in the body, their physical benefits differ.

Every movement that your muscles make draws on reserves of energy. In order to meet this demand, your body must continually replenish the energy stores of the muscles. Energy can be supplied to the muscles using one or more of three systems: the phosphocreatine, the lactic acid, or the aerobic. Which one comes into play depends on the intensity and duration of the exercise being undertaken.

Highly exertive exercise performed for three minutes or less—sprinting, for example, demands that your body use the first two forms of energy production, the phosphocreatine and the lactic acid, neither of which requires oxygen. Together they are known as the anaerobic (without oxygen) systems. Low-intensity exercise that lasts for more than three minutes draws on a form of energy production involving oxygen. This is the aerobic (with oxygen) system. When your muscles are at rest, even though they are never totally inactive, their energy reserves are topped up at a steady rate from all three systems.

ANAEROBIC SYSTEMS

Anaerobic systems can deliver energy very quickly; thus they provide the power needed for short bursts of sudden activity, for instance, jumping out of a chair and dashing upstairs. Energy provided anaerobically is quickly used up by the body, however, so these systems cannot maintain the fuel supplies needed for sustained exercise, such as a 20-minute run.

AEROBIC VERSUS ANAEROBIC EXERCISE

Having a good general level of fitness means undertaking both aerobic and anaerobic exercise. Aerobic exercise helps to improve overall cardiovascular fitness, whereas anaerobic exercise helps to build strength. The amount of each form of exercise that you do depends on your current fitness level and exercise goals.

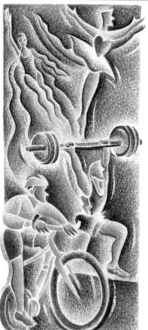

DIFFERENT TYPES OF EXERCISE	ADVANTAGES	DISADVANTAGES
Aerobic exercise includes walking, jogging, cycling, and swimming, which can be sustained for long periods.	Level of intensity can gradually be increased, making this suitable for all fitness levels. Improves cardiovascular function, a basic measure of fitness. Medium-intensity aerobic exercise utilizes fat as an energy source, making it useful as part of a weight reduction program.	Exercise must be sustained for at least 20 minutes and performed regularly to be effective.
Anaerobic exercise includes weight lifting, sprinting, ballet lifts, and sports like hockey, all of which require sudden, intense movements.	Can help build strength and power to carry out everyday activities. Increased strength leads to lower risk of injury. Increased speed, strength, and power improve ability to enjoy sports.	Requires a high level of fitness. Can place sudden strain on the body. Lactic acid produced as side effect causes pain and fatigue.

Phosphocreatine

This system is the first to be drawn on for energy. It breaks down a high-energy storage molecule called phosphocreatine, which is held in the muscles. It is very responsive to the muscles' needs for energy and is capable of supplying large amounts of energy very quickly but lasts only a brief time. For example, it will supply the energy used when a person runs for a bus.

The phosphocreatine system is sometimes thought of as the start-up system. Like the battery of a car, which supplies a sudden burst of energy to start the engine, it provides a sudden burst of energy to set the muscles moving. The system is also called upon when high-intensity activity demands more energy than the other energy systems can meet, for instance, when a person is sprinting or lifting an extremely heavy weight. Also like the car battery, the phosphocreatine system can become drained quickly. Just as running a car at a steady pace for a while will utilize energy from the fuel system to recharge the battery, in the same way energy produced aerobically recharges the phosphocreatine system.

In general, stored phosphocreatine has the capacity to supply the body with enough energy to walk quickly for about 1 minute, to run for 20 to 30 seconds, or to sprint flat out for 6 seconds.

Lactic acid

Carbohydrate is stored as glycogen in the liver and muscles. The lactic acid system breaks down glycogen to release energy. This is the best form of energy for more sustained periods of high-intensity activity because, unlike the aerobic system, it is not

ENERGY PRODUCTION SYSTEMS

The energy to power muscles can come either from processes that do not use oxygen, called anaerobic systems, or from one that does, the aerobic system. The anaerobic systems quickly supply high-intensity energy but cannot sustain it for long periods. The aerobic system, on the other hand, supplies low-intensity, sustainable energy. One of the anaerobic systems produces the waste product lactic acid, which builds up to the point at which muscular activity is no longer possible. Once the high-intensity activity stops, oxygen can be made available to remove the lactic acid by converting it into glucose and carbon dioxide.

ANAEROBIC SYSTEMS (WITHOUT OXYGEN)

AEROBIC SYSTEM (WITH OXYGEN)

PHOSPHOCREATINE SYSTEM

Phospho-creatine is broken down to release rapid energy.

Energy produced is of high intensity but short duration.

LACTIC ACID SYSTEM

Glycogen is broken down to release more energy along with unwanted **lactic acid.**

Lactic acid buildup causes pain and fatigue.

Glycogen and fatty acids are broken down using **oxygen.**

Energy produced is of low intensity but can be sustained.

ENERGY FOR SPRINT RACES
A sprint race requires anaerobic energy because the blood cannot supply oxygen fast enough for the aerobic system to operate. The waste product lactic acid builds up in the muscles, causing fatigue and pain until it is impossible to go on.

ENERGY FOR DISTANCE RACES
A distance race is of lower intensity, so oxygen can be supplied fast enough for the aerobic system to work. The waste product carbon dioxide is easily removed from the body.

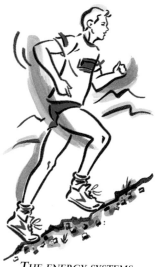

THE ENERGY SYSTEMS
A sequence like running at a steady pace for 20 minutes, then jogging up a hill for 30 seconds, and then sprinting for 1 minute requires shifting between the three different energy systems. The aerobic system is used for the constant, moderate endurance phase; the phosphocreatine system is called on for the high-energy hill climb; and the lactic acid system comes into play for the quick minute of sprint power.

limited by the speed at which the blood circulation can supply oxygen to the muscles in order to operate. However, in breaking down, glycogen releases lactate, which builds up in the muscles in the form of the waste product lactic acid. Lactic acid build-up blocks muscle contraction, causing a burning sensation and pain. This acts as a safety valve, forcing the body to slow down or stop when the intensity is too great. At high intensities it takes between 45 seconds and 3 minutes for lactic acid to accumulate to a level that causes pain.

Although the lactic acid system is anaerobic, once we stop high-intensity exercise, oxygen is required in a process that removes lactic acid by breaking it down into glucose and carbon dioxide. This requirement is called the oxygen debt and is the reason that we pant for breath after sprinting.

THE AEROBIC SYSTEM

The aerobic system takes over the task of supplying energy to the muscles when exercise is sustained for longer periods. Aerobic fitness describes the body's ability to take in, transport, and use oxygen to meet the energy demands of the muscles. Improved aerobic fitness allows you to carry out moderate-intensity exercise for longer periods of time with less effort.

Both carbohydrate and fat are broken down in the aerobic system in a process involving oxygen; this is called oxidation. The oxidation of carbohydrate in the form of glycogen supplies most of your energy needs. Low-intensity exercise of long duration, however, relies much more on fat as a fuel. Although fat is a very dense energy source—1 gram of fat supplies about 9 calories of energy—its breakdown requires large amounts of oxygen, which limits the intensity of exercise that it can fuel. This is why more intense exercise is fueled by carbohydrate breakdown and phosphocreatine.

CHOOSING AN EXERCISE TO MAKE YOU FIT

The question of which form of exercise is best for promoting fitness depends on the individual's definition of fit, which can mean many things to many people. To one person it may mean carrying out everyday tasks without requiring help. To others it may mean being able to go windsurfing, cycling, or hiking every weekend without feeling tired and sore or performing well in competition in their chosen sport.

Whichever definition is applied, attaining fitness involves a mixture of anaerobic and aerobic activities. The decisions people make about what they want to achieve by being fit will determine the balance of anaerobic activities (high intensity) and aerobic activities (low to moderate intensity) in their chosen exercise program.

A sprinter will need mainly high-intensity activity, whereas a marathon runner will need a greater mix of low- and moderate-intensity activities. For general improvements in health, a buildup from low to moderate intensity is recommended.

HIGH OR LOW INTENSITY?

Some people think that only high-intensity exercise promotes true physical fitness. However, a California study produced some surprising results. Three groups of men and women aged 50 to 60, all of whom had previously been sedentary, were given exercise programs to do at different levels of intensity. The first group did high-intensity exercise in a class; the second did high-intensity exercise at home; and the third did lower-intensity exercise at home. All three groups significantly improved their fitness level, regardless of the intensity of their workouts.

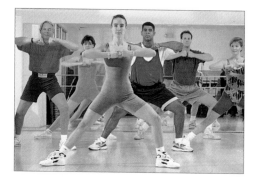

GETTING THE BALANCE RIGHT
Finding the right balance of high- and low-intensity exercise depends on your goals. In most cases low to moderate intensity is best.

COMPONENTS OF FITNESS

All-round fitness involves three components—stamina, strength, and flexibility. To achieve your fitness goals, you may need to concentrate more on some areas than on others.

When you begin a new fitness program, it is important to give some thought to what you want to achieve, that is, which aspects of your fitness and health you wish to improve. If your sole concern is to lose some weight, then an intense course of strength training alone will not help you achieve this, whereas a low-fat diet combined with regular aerobic exercise and some exercises to improve strength will produce a clearly noticeable difference in a matter of weeks. Most people find that they have strengths and weaknesses in different areas, and they must take these into account when they plan an exercise program.

STAMINA

Stamina has a variety of names, including cardiovascular endurance, cardiopulmonary endurance, and aerobic fitness. All these terms refer to the capacity of the heart and lungs to supply oxygen to the working muscles and the ability of the muscles to extract that oxygen and use it to release energy from stored carbohydrate and fat.

With regular stamina training, the body develops stronger, more elastic blood vessels and a bigger, stronger heart that is able to pump a larger volume of blood with each beat. This improves the blood supply both to the heart itself and to the muscles around the body that are being worked.

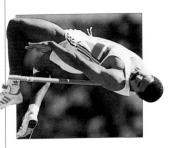

MASTER OF THE DECATHLON
The decathlon, which involves 10 different events, requires stamina, strength, and flexibility. This means that competitors must excel in all aspects of physical fitness. In the 1980s the decathlon world record holder, Daley Thompson, was called "the world's greatest all-round athlete."

CROSS TRAINING

Crosstraining involves working on all the components of fitness in one session by doing aerobic exercises, strength training, and stretches. This provides a thorough workout and brings variety to a routine, which helps maintain interest. The amount of each type of exercise you do depends on your personal goals.

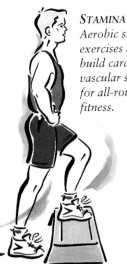

STAMINA
Aerobic step exercises help build cardiovascular stamina for all-round fitness.

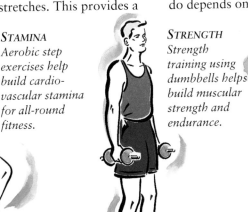

STRENGTH
Strength training using dumbbells helps build muscular strength and endurance.

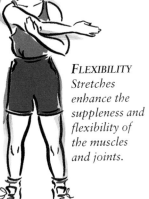

FLEXIBILITY
Stretches enhance the suppleness and flexibility of the muscles and joints.

Belly dancing for muscular strength

You don't have to use weights to build muscular strength and endurance. Belly dancing, for example, is good for developing both muscular strength and flexibility, especially in the abdominal and lower back muscles. It is also great fun to do, and you don't need a high level of fitness to begin with.

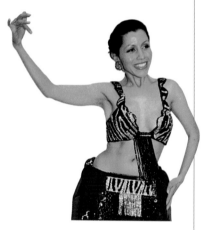

DANCE OF THE EAST
Belly dancing originated in the Middle East but is becoming increasingly popular in the West, where it is taught in evening classes and community centers, as well as dance schools.

WORKING AT THE CORRECT INTENSITY

This table shows how to use your own responses to judge the intensity of your exercise. If you are a beginner, you should train at levels 1 and 2, which will leave you only slightly breathless. If you are already active, you should train at levels 1 and 2 but also include some exercise at level 3, which should make you breathless but still able to talk. Athletes usually train at all levels of intensity.

Level 1	Easy—I could keep going at this level for a long time.
Level 2	I am slightly breathless but can still keep going at this level.
Level 3	I am somewhat breathless but can still manage to talk.
Level 4	I am so breathless that I don't want to talk anymore.
Level 5	I couldn't talk even if I tried.

Stamina training improves lung capacity, increasing the volume of air that is moved in and out of the lungs with each breath. It also improves the body's ability to extract oxygen from the air, resulting in easier breathing at any level of exertion.

Forms of stamina training

Any form of aerobic exercise will enhance your stamina. Brisk walking, swimming, skating, jogging, running, cycling, dancing, rowing, and aerobic step and dance routines are all effective. Chapter 7 looks at home exercises you can try and illustrates an aerobic routine that can be done anywhere to improve cardiovascular fitness.

Training intensity

The intensity of stamina training is directly related to heart rate. Your maximum heart rate potential is the uppermost level at which your heart should be able to beat during exercise; this varies according to age.

A safe way to estimate your maximum heart rate—number of beats per minute—is to subtract your age from 220. For a 30-year-old man, for example, this would be 220 minus 30, which equals 190; thus 190 is his maximum heart rate.

A newcomer to exercise should start training at a lower intensity—around 65 percent of maximum heart rate (see page 61). Healthy people who exercise regularly can train at up to 85 percent of their maximum heart rate. Only serious athletes, particularly those involved in competitive sports, need to include some exercise activity at 85 to 90 percent of maximum heart rate in their training program.

Training duration

When training to improve stamina, the same benefits can be gained from carrying out low-intensity activities of longer duration as from more vigorous activities of shorter duration. Current medical opinion recommends that for improved health we should do at least 20 minutes of moderate-intensity activity, such as brisk walking, a minimum of three times a week. For greater aerobic fitness, however, longer periods of a more vigorous activity, such as running, three or more times a week is necessary.

MUSCULAR STRENGTH AND ENDURANCE

At its most basic level, strength and endurance training ensures that muscles are able to meet the physical demands that normal activity puts on them, such as getting in and out of the bathtub, carrying shopping bags, and maintaining good posture, without getting unduly fatigued or sustaining injury. It can also help ensure that you maintain a good level of strength throughout your life.

Weight training is the best-known type of strength and endurance training, but it conjures up images of competitive bodybuilders, which can be off-putting to many people. However, strength and endurance can be achieved through many other forms of exercise, including dance.

Benefits of strength training

The health benefits of strength training include reducing the risk of serious injury, making it easier to carry out everyday activities, and improving your resting metabolic rate and body composition. It also increases or maintains bone density, depending on your age, which reduces the risk of osteoporosis in later life.

However, if you have high blood pressure, you should seek medical advice before starting high-intensity weight training because it can increase blood pressure to unsafe levels.

Isometric and isotonic movements

In any activity some muscles will be causing movement while others will be checking movement in order to stabilize the body. The muscles causing movement are working isotonically, and those checking movement are working isometrically. Take care when training isometrically, such as supporting a heavy weight or your own body weight for several seconds without moving, as this increases blood pressure dramatically.

Strength training without weights

Muscular strength and endurance training can be carried out without weights. One method is callisthenics, which involves gymnastic exercises that boost strength and encourage graceful movement. Many techniques used in aerobic step or circuit training also increase strength and endurance.

Muscles must be pushed beyond their previous levels in order to stimulate them to improve. They can be worked with the same weight, or resistance, but for a longer duration in order to improve muscular endurance, or with a greater weight but the same duration to improve strength.

FLEXIBILITY AND STRETCHING

Flexibility is crucial to ensure a complete range of movement, good posture, reduced muscle stiffness, and lower risk of injury. The key to developing and keeping flexibility is to stretch often. However, stretches should be performed only after the muscles of the body are warmed up. In sports that involve a lot of stretching, such as swimming, it is important to warm up and do stretching exercises before participating.

Active and passive stretching

There are two main types of stretching: active and passive. Active stretches are movements in which one muscle is extended while its opposing muscle is contracted. Active stretching performs two exercise functions at once: it develops the flexibility of the muscle being stretched and strengthens the muscle being contracted.

Passive stretching occurs when gravity or some other outside influence exerts pressure to stretch the target muscle. This is a safe way of stretching because it does not involve any sudden movement. Performed gradually, it gives the muscles and connective tissue time to adapt to the stretch.

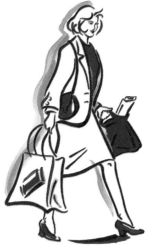

*MUSCLE MOVEMENT
When you walk and carry an object, such as a bag, the muscles in your legs work isotonically—propelling you forward—while the muscles of your torso and arms work isometrically—keeping you upright and supporting the bag.*

FLEXIBILITY AND STRETCHING

Flexibility and stretching movements should be performed before exercise to warm and stretch the muscles; after exercise, when the muscles are warm and can be lengthened more easily; and at any time during the day to revive yourself and stay supple.

***ACTIVE STRETCHING**
An example of active stretching is to stand up straight and reach toward the ceiling. In this instance the shoulder muscles contract in order to stretch (extend) the large muscles of the upper back.*

***PASSIVE STRETCHING**
An example of passive stretching is sitting on the floor with your legs straight out in front of you, then leaning forward. This stretches the muscles at the back of the leg (hamstrings) and in the lower back.*

PNF
Proprioceptive neuromuscular facilitation, PNF for short, is an advanced form of stretching used by athletes and therapists to increase range of motion. It involves alternately stretching, contracting, and relaxing a muscle and is more easily carried out with a partner.

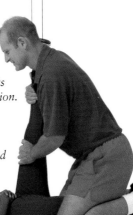

HOW MUCH EXERCISE AND WHEN?

Lack of physical activity is known to be a contributing factor to many diseases in the West. Research has been done to find out just how much exercise is needed to maintain good health.

TIME VERSUS INTENSITY
When selecting an activity to help you stay fit, look for one that you enjoy and that fits readily into your day. Moderate physical activity is roughly defined as using about 150 calories of energy during the time spent doing it; each of the activities below fits this criterion. Remember that the less vigorous the exercise is, the more time you must spend at it in order to burn up the same number of calories.

Medical experts throughout the world have been issuing statements regarding the amount of physical activity necessary to keep a person fit and healthy. Many of these concentrate on cardiovascular activity, though more recent reports also focus on the benefits of muscular strength and endurance.

HOW OFTEN?
All health researchers agree that physical inactivity is a precursor to ill health and, in particular, a major contributing factor to cardiovascular disease. Doctors now recommend that exercise be performed on a regular basis to help prevent a wide range of illnesses. Everyone should try to get in as much exercise as possible throughout the week, working at a level appropriate to individual needs and capabilities.

Twenty minutes or more of moderate exercise at least three times a week is the recommended minimum amount for all children and adults to live a healthier lifestyle. This amount of exercise will maintain cardiovascular health and aerobic fitness. If you already exercise at this level, you can gain additional benefits by becoming even more active or by increasing the intensity of your workouts. In any case, it is advisable, particularly for older people, to be active every day in some way, even if it is just just walking around the neighborhood.

No particular exercise or sport can be singled out as a more effective way to get fit; any one you choose will work, as long as it is performed at an intensity that raises and sustains your metabolic rate for the entire duration. In short, whatever exercise, activity, or sport you participate in will be beneficial.

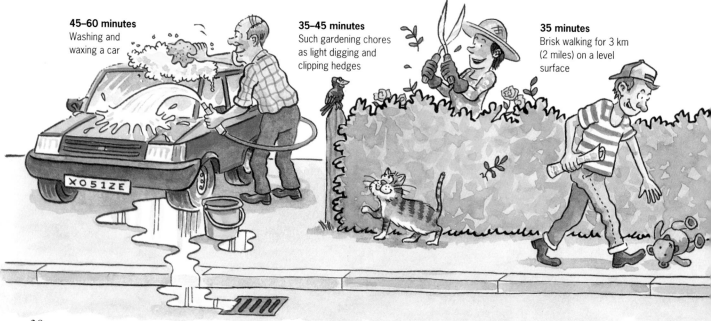

45–60 minutes
Washing and waxing a car

35–45 minutes
Such gardening chores as light digging and clipping hedges

35 minutes
Brisk walking for 3 km (2 miles) on a level surface

CHOOSING THE BEST TIME TO EXERCISE

At whatever time you can fit exercise into your routine and feel comfortable doing it is the best time to schedule it. This may be before or after work, while the children are at school, or at lunchtime. The most important thing is to exercise on a regular basis.

Some people need the stimulation of working out at different times of the day and varying their regimen to avoid becoming bored and abandoning their exercise goals. Others thrive on routine. If they establish a habit of going to a gym or jogging at a particular time on certain days, exercise becomes a habit and they don't have to struggle with the effort of fitting it into their life. Whatever the approach, most people who exercise regularly find that they miss it when they aren't able to do it.

Vigorous exercise is not advisable immediately after a heavy meal because stomach cramps may result. Light exercise, like a stroll, after a meal can be beneficial, however, as it has been shown to increase the uptake and usage of fat by the muscles.

Exercising vigorously or for long periods without eating is not advisable either, because muscles become depleted of carbohydrates, leading to fatigue, loss of power, and perhaps light-headedness and an inability to concentrate. Vigorous exercise is usually more effective if undertaken later in the day, after you have had time to digest a meal and your body has had time to wake up. If you do exercise early in the morning, have a low-glycemic food (see page 46) beforehand.

During exercise of long duration, such as a full day of hiking or cycling, the muscles need to be refueled at regular intervals with high-carbohydrate foods. It is possible to eat something and carry on with the activity right away, as long as the exercise is at a low intensity for the period right after eating and the food is one that is easily digested.

For beginners short bouts of 10 to 15 minutes of exercise carried out several times a day are usually easier to cope with than one longer exercise session.

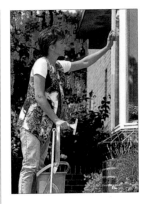

HIDDEN EXERCISE OPPORTUNITIES
There are many ways to exercise without donning gym shorts or a sweat suit. Window washing, for example, can build muscle, stamina, and flexibility, especially when it involves moving and climbing a ladder. Other household chores that involve bending, stretching, and/or lifting are also good exercise.

Pathway to health

The more you exercise, the more important it is to eat well balanced meals that supply sufficient calories, or you will find yourself becoming fatigued. In addition, you must drink plenty of liquid every time you exercise to replace fluids lost through sweat, whether or not you are thirsty. You may become dangerously dehydrated otherwise.

Safe exercise also entails resting any strained muscles. The old adage "no pain, no gain" is not something to aim for because it is likely to result in injury. If you feel pain, stop. If pain persists for more than two days after an injury, see your doctor.

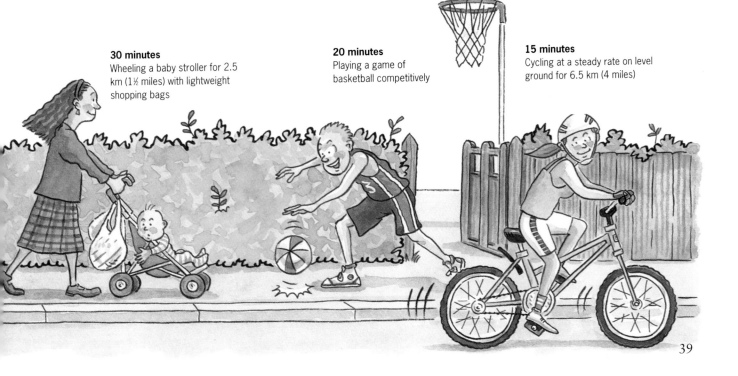

30 minutes
Wheeling a baby stroller for 2.5 km (1½ miles) with lightweight shopping bags

20 minutes
Playing a game of basketball competitively

15 minutes
Cycling at a steady rate on level ground for 6.5 km (4 miles)

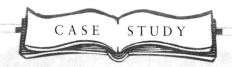

A Woman with Hypertension

*Being overweight is often a cause of hypertension, or high blood pressure.
Couple this with a sedentary lifestyle, and the ramifications can be even more serious.
Cutting back on high-fat foods and those high in cholesterol is a step in the right
direction, but for maximum benefit regular exercise is also needed.*

Sarah is 48 years old and married with two teenage children. She works as a secretary in a busy office just five minutes from her house. After a recent routine checkup, her doctor said that her blood pressure was too high. Sarah currently does no exercise at all and is overweight. She eats well-balanced meals during the day but tends to nibble on high-sugar, high-fat snacks in the evening while she watches television. After Sarah described her daily regimen, the doctor told her that in order to lose weight and lower her blood pressure, all she needed to do was moderate her snacking in the evenings and take up some form of low-impact aerobic exercise. Ideally, Sarah should exercise two or three times a week to begin with.

WHAT SHOULD SARAH DO?

Sarah needs to find an activity that she will enjoy and that will fit into her lifestyle without too much disruption. If she exercises in the evening, she will have the added bonus of occupying some of the time she now spends watching television and snacking.

Because Sarah enjoyed swimming when she was in college, a good option for her would be to take it up again. However, she will find that she isn't capable of doing as much as she used to and will have to build up the intensity and length of her swims gradually. Sarah must also cut out the high-sugar and high-fat snacks and replace them with healthy options, such as fruit or raw vegetables with low-fat dips.

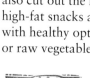

LIFESTYLE
A sedentary lifestyle can quickly lead to weight gain and lack of fitness.

FITNESS
Lack of regular exercise contributes to obesity and high blood pressure, as well as many other diseases and general poor health.

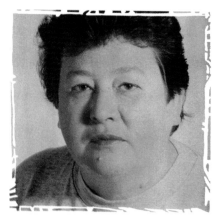

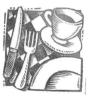

DIET
Frequent high-fat, high-sugar snacks can quickly pile on the calories.

Action Plan

LIFESTYLE
Find ways to introduce exercise into everyday life, such as taking a walk at lunchtime instead of sitting in the cafeteria.

FITNESS
Exercise for 30 minutes a couple of nights a week to begin with, gradually building this up to three or more sessions a week.

DIET
Allow snacks only one day a week while watching television. Limit snacks for the rest of the week or choose healthy options instead, such as nonfat crackers or fruit.

HOW THINGS TURNED OUT FOR SARAH

As Sarah's confidence in the water returned, she found that she was still quite a good swimmer, and she now visits the pool regularly. She managed to wean herself off the unhealthy snacks with surprising ease, and they are now only an occasional indulgence. After three months Sarah had lost 6.5 kilos (14 pounds), and a checkup by her doctor showed that her blood pressure was back within acceptable levels.

CHOOSING A HEALTHY ACTIVITY

Taking up a sport or other physical pursuit that you enjoy is a good way to enhance your health and fitness and at the same time remain motivated to stay with an exercise regimen.

All sports and other active leisure pursuits provide their own unique combination of health benefits. Some activities, such as chess or fishing, promote relaxation and stress relief but do little to improve aspects of physical conditioning. Some activities enhance a particular physical attribute, such as speed, strength, or flexibility, while others provide a mixture of them.

By taking part in two or three different pursuits rather than concentrating on one, you can gain a wide range of health benefits. If you prefer to limit yourself to a single pursuit, you can still maintain all-round physical fitness by training for those components of fitness that are not developed by your chosen activity. For example, cyclists could do some strength and endurance exercises for their upper body. Players of racquet sports could add strength and endurance work for the arm that does not hold the racquet. Distance runners could include strength exercises and some flexibility training in their regimen.

If you have not been active for some time, you should work up to your maximum output gradually, building up your time and intensity according to your capabilities. Suddenly playing badminton for an hour or walking briskly for 5 kilometers (3 miles) will give you sore muscles and possibly discourage you from taking part again. How quickly you become comfortable in a new activity or get back into a sport you once

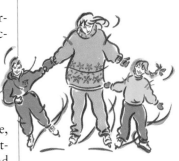

FUN ON ICE
Ice skating can be enjoyed at all levels, from an occasional visit to the rink with family and friends to daily training sessions to reach competition standards.

WHAT IS SPORT?

Some people have a restrictive view of sports, tending to picture stereotypes of highly competitive athletes. Interestingly, the dictionary defines *sport* not only as "a game or competitive activity involving physical exertion" but also as "a source of diversion or fun." A sport can be a form of artistic expression as well. For example, gymnastic floor exercises, ice skating, dancing, and synchronized swimming are activities that involve a high level of artistry. When thinking about sport options, consider your personal likes and dislikes and your temperament. Sports can offer you the chance to express your creativity, challenge your skill, give you opportunities to socialize, or provide you with time for relaxation and reflection.

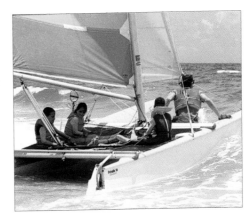

GET FIT TO HAVE FUN
Training for and taking part in a sport throughout the year will keep you fit enough to take advantage of an active holiday pursuit that may arise unexpectedly, such as the opportunity to spend a day sailing.

enjoyed will depend on your age, the number of years you have been inactive, and your psychological makeup.

THE FUN OF COMPETITION

Many people are attracted to activities that involve intense competition with other persons, whereas others prefer to compete against the elements or against themselves. Few ramblers or hikers would consider themselves in any competition. Rather, their achievement is in finishing the walk or hike and perhaps scrambling over rough terrain or up and down steep hills.

Likewise, many marathon runners take part in events knowing that they will never win the race, but are content to compete against themselves, striving to improve their personal best time. Members of sports teams continue to turn out week after week and strive to do their best because they enjoy the game, even after a long run of losses has ruled out any likelihood of a trophy. In choosing a sport, the aim should be to compete at a level that will extend your abilities a little but is not so demanding that you become discouraged.

Any leisure pursuit can be made competitive for those who prefer it. Some health clubs have ultra-fit competitions, and ballroom dancers compete all over the world. Challenge walking involves completing set routes, varying from a few kilometers to many hundreds of kilometers, within a time limit. There is no prize for finishing first, and the last person home is as much a winner as the first. The competition is between the individual and the conditions. Some cycling events provide the same challenge. Participants still have to train, however, to make sure that they are fit enough to complete the event.

For many people competitive sports provide the incentive to train regularly and increase their activity level beyond the minimum necessary for health. In some sports it is the training, rather than the competition, that can be of particular value to health.

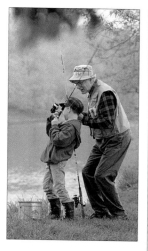

GONE FISHING
Fishing can be very beneficial for reducing stress and promoting relaxation. It can also build fitness if a fair amount of walking is involved.

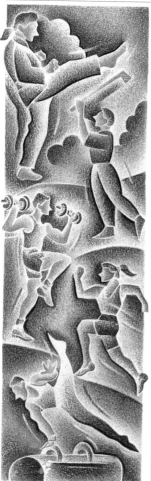

FITNESS COMPONENTS OF DIFFERENT ACTIVITIES

Choosing a sport or exercise to take up can initially be a daunting task. However, if you know what areas of fitness you want to develop, the table below can help you decide which is the right sport or exercise for you.

SPORT	MUSCULAR STRENGTH	AEROBIC STAMINA	MUSCULAR STAMINA	FLEXIBILITY
Aerobics		✔	✔	✔
Dancing	✔	✔	✔	✔
Circuit training	✔	✔	✔	✔
Walking		✔	✔	
Running		✔	✔	
Rowing	✔	✔	✔	✔
Swimming	✔	✔	✔	✔
Martial arts	✔		✔	✔
Downhill skiing		✔	✔	✔
Gymnastics	✔		✔	✔
Racquet sports		✔	✔	✔
Golf		✔	✔	
Cycling		✔	✔	

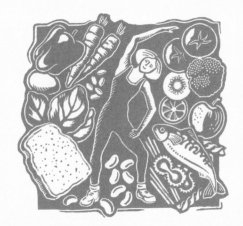

CHAPTER 3

EXERCISE AND DIET

An exercise program will bring the most benefits if it is underpinned by a healthy diet. To perform effectively during exercise, your body needs the right food, in the right amounts, at the right time. Exactly what this right diet is can vary for different forms of exercise.

COMBINING EXERCISE AND DIET

One of the most important requirements for exercising effectively is to make sure that your body receives the correct fuel to sustain your chosen activities.

THE RIGHT COMBINATION
To maximize exercise performance and ensure good health, the bulk of your diet should be made up of grain products (preferably whole grain), followed by fruits and vegetables. Low-fat dairy products and protein foods such as meat, fish, legumes, and eggs should comprise the next largest constituents; the smallest percentage should be fats and refined sugars.

The energy you need for exercising effectively comes from converting the food you eat into the fuel that powers your body. To understand your energy needs for exercise you must first comprehend your body's basic daily requirements and how exercise increases them.

THE BASICS OF HEALTHY EATING

Everyone should be aware of the basic elements of healthy eating. Once understood, these can then be adapted to suit specific exercise needs. The most important aspect of a healthful diet is getting the right balance of the various food elements.

Carbohydrates—both simple and complex—supply the basic fuel your body needs, so foods high in carbohydrate should form the largest part of your diet—55 to 65 percent. Simple carbohydrates, or sugars, are prevalent in fruit. Good sources of complex carbohydrates, or starches, include bread, rice, pasta, and breakfast cereals.

Protein, which should comprise 10 to 15 percent of daily calories, is needed for growth, repair, and replacement of body tissues, such as muscle, and the manufacture of hormones and enzymes. Good sources of protein include meat, fish, poultry, eggs, dairy products, and legumes, such as peas, beans, peanuts, soybeans, and lentils.

Fats also supply energy, but these should comprise no more than 30 percent of your diet and preferably less. There are two kinds of dietary fat, saturated—the predominant kind in meat, egg yolks, and whole-milk foods—and unsaturated—found largely in nuts, seeds, and oily fish. Saturated fat should be limited to 10 percent of a daily diet because it can raise cholesterol levels and lead to clogged arteries.

Oily fish, like tuna and salmon, and some plant oils—corn, safflower, and flaxseed, for example—also contain essential fatty acids (EFAs), which cannot be manufactured by the body. Foods containing EFAs should be eaten in small amounts every day.

Your diet should also contain ample fiber, which is mainly obtained from whole-grain cereal products, fruits, and vegetables. There are two types. Insoluble fiber, also known as roughage, absorbs water and provides the bulk needed to carry waste products through the body quickly. Soluble fiber prevents the digestive system from reabsorbing fats and helps keep cholesterol levels low. Insufficient fiber has been linked to health problems, including chronic constipation.

For optimum health nutritionists recommend that you have 5 to 10 servings of fruits and vegetables every day. In addition to being rich sources of carbohydrates and fiber, these foods provide many of the vitamins, minerals, and other nutrients essential for the healthy functioning of your body.

Drink plenty of water every day too—at least eight glasses. Water carries nutrients throughout the body, lubricates joints, and aids digestion and absorption of food. A diet based on the above principles will

RAISING METABOLIC RATE THROUGH REGULAR EXERCISE

Regular exercise makes the heart and lungs work more efficiently and increases muscle mass; as a result, you burn more energy (calories) and your metabolic rate goes up. To maintain a steady weight, your daily calorie intake must match energy output. The charts below show the recommended calorie intake for men and women according to their level of activity. (To convert weight in pounds to kilograms, divide by 2.2.)

▨ **Male**   ▨ **Female**

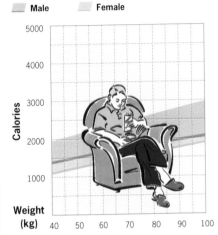

SEDENTARY LIFESTYLE
When you are mainly inactive, your heart and lungs are less efficient and you have little muscle growth, so your metabolic rate remains low.

REGULAR EXERCISE
Once you start to exercise regularly, your heart rate rises, your lungs work harder, your muscles increase in size, and your metabolic rate rises.

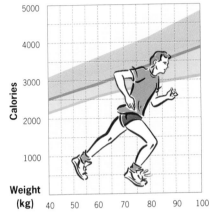

INCREASED EXERCISE
When you follow a fitness routine, your heart and lungs work more efficiently, your muscles burn more calories, and your metabolic rate rises even more.

ensure that you have all the essential nutrients for good health. Exercise, however, places extra demands on your body that may require some changes in your diet.

BASAL METABOLIC RATE

Basal metabolic rate (BMR) is the amount of energy needed for such basic physiological processes as breathing, circulation of blood, and heartbeat. This is separate from the energy required for activities like walking and dancing. The BMR accounts for the largest proportion of total daily energy expenditure—up to 75 percent in people who are mainly sedentary.

BMR is determined by many factors, including genetic makeup, age, sex, and body size and composition. Men tend to have a higher BMR than women because they have a higher proportion of muscle tissue to fat. Muscle is metabolically active—that is, it burns calories even when you are at rest—so increases in muscle mass that result from exercise are reflected in an increase in BMR.

Periods of energy imbalance or a shortage of calories can trigger a drop in BMR. This is an important consideration when assessing your food intake because your body will attempt to overcome any shortfall in calories by conserving energy, which may leave you feeling tired and lethargic.

Activity and metabolism

Any activity raises your energy expenditure and metabolic rate above BMR. Washing, ironing, even sitting and reading will have an effect, but the increase is more dramatic with such energetic exercise as running or cycling. Activity levels can vary dramatically from person to person and from day to day in the same person, but in someone who is primarily sedentary, activity above BMR accounts for between 15 and 30 percent of total daily energy expenditure. In athletes this figure can rise to 50 percent.

The most important factor affecting the metabolic rate is the intensity of exercise; the increase will become more pronounced as the intensity of training increases. Increasing your level of activity may require an increase in food intake to maintain your present weight—not only because you are using more energy but also because, over time, regular exercise raises your BMR and

MUSCLE MATTERS
You do not have to lift heavy weights to develop more muscle. Such activities as dancing and swimming will also increase muscle bulk.

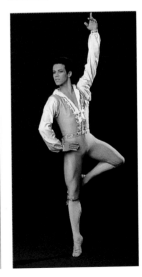

GLYCEMIC INDEX

The foods below on the left, higher on the glycemic index (GI), provide quick energy for intense exercise. Those on the right, lower on the GI, release energy more slowly for sustained exercise. All are compared to glucose, which equals 100 on the index.

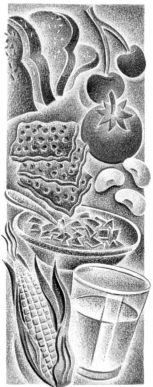

HIGHER GI FOODS		
FOOD GROUP	FOOD ITEM	NUMBER
Grains	Macaroni & cheese	64
	Rice, brown	59
	Rice cakes	77
Breakfast cereals	Cornflakes	83
	Oatmeal (quick)	66
	Rice squares	89
Bread, Crackers	Whole-wheat bread	72
	Crisp bread, rye	63
	Saltines	72
Vegetables	Beets	64
	Potato, baked	85
	Potato, french-fried	75
Fruits	Banana, ripe	62
	Raisins	64

LOWER GI FOODS		
FOOD GROUP	FOOD ITEM	NUMBER
Fruits, juices	Apples	38
	Apricots, dried	30
	Cherries	22
	Grapes	43
	Pineapple juice	46
Legumes	Baked beans, canned	48
	Chickpeas	33
	Soybeans	18
Dairy products	Ice cream, low-fat	50
	Milk, skim	32
	Milk, whole	27
	Yogurt, low-fat, fruit	33
	Yogurt, low-fat, plain	38
Soup	Tomato	38

you expend more energy even when resting. It's a good idea to look carefully at your current diet, as well as the fuel demands of your exercise routine, to see whether you need to make any dietary changes.

ENERGY REQUIREMENTS DURING EXERCISE

When you embark on an exercise program, you should match your nutritional intake to the energy demands being made on the body and the expected increase in your basal metabolic rate. An increase in BMR is mainly a result of the extra muscle mass you develop during exercise. If you are not getting sufficient calories to satisfy these needs, you will lose weight (perhaps a desired goal), but you may also become fatigued if the balance of nutrients is not right.

Carbohydrates, fat, and protein all provide fuel for exercise, but only carbohydrates and fat play significant roles. Which fuel is burned during exercise depends on many factors, including the intensity, duration, and training status. As exercise becomes more intense, there is a greater reliance on carbohydrates, but as the duration increases, there is a reduction in the role that carbohydrates play in providing energy and an increase in the contribution from fat.

CARBOHYDRATE

Carbohydrate is the major fuel used for exercise, particularly intense exercise, but body stores are limited to about 300 grams in sedentary people and up to 500 grams in trained athletes. Energy from carbohydrate is released within exercising muscles up to three times faster than the energy from fat. Carbohydrate from food is converted by the body into glucose and glycogen, the long-term storage form of glucose. Glycogen is held in the liver and muscles, where it is quickly converted into glucose when needed.

When glucose becomes depleted, fatigue sets in, and the liver compensates by converting more glycogen into glucose to restore the balance. To maximize glycogen storage, it is important to eat adequate amounts of carbohydrate. Current recommendations are that sedentary people eat a minimum of 4.5 grams of carbohydrate per kilogram of body weight per day. For someone weighing 63.5 kilograms (140 pounds) this would mean an intake of about 285 grams of carbohydrate per day. (The largest proportion should come from complex carbohydrates, preferably whole-grain ones.) Athletes in training require about twice this amount, or 8 to 9 grams of carbohydrate per kilogram of body weight each day.

The speed at which the carbohydrates in different foods break down to provide glucose for the body is classified on a scale known as the glycemic index, or GI (see opposite page). The number after each food indicates the effect it has on blood glucose levels for one to two hours after it is eaten. Foods with a higher rating break down quickly; those with a lower one take longer, supplying glucose to the bloodstream slowly.

Many complex carbohydrates, such as pasta and legumes, have a low GI. This is because they have to be broken down into a simple form of carbohydrate before they can be used to provide energy. Foods that contain a higher proportion of simple carbohydrates, on the other hand, such as raisins and carrots, rate higher on the GI because they reach the bloodstream more quickly and thus offer a rapid energy source.

However, the equation is not simply one of complex carbohydrates having a low GI value and simple carbohydrates having a high one. Fruits, for instance, are mainly simple carbohydrates but they also contain fiber, which slows their rate of digestion and absorption. They have a lower GI and act more like a complex carbohydrate.

FAT

Fat is the body's principal energy reserve. It is stored mainly in the muscles and as adipose tissue around the body. Fat is broken down into free fatty acids (FFAs), which can be released for use as an energy source to fuel muscles during exercise. They are stored as triglycerides in fat cells and in muscle fibers to be used by the muscles after being broken down.

The rate at which triglycerides are broken down may, in part, determine the rate at which muscles use fat as fuel during exercise. More oxygen is required to release energy from fat than from carbohydrate, and there appears to be a metabolic limit to the ability of fat to generate energy, so fat alone cannot be used to sustain exercise at higher levels of intensity. While even the leanest athletes have enough fat stored within their bodies to exercise for long periods, they simply cannot convert all of it for effective use during intensive exercise and must rely on their carbohydrate reserves.

PROTEIN

Protein is essential for many of the body's vital functions, including tissue repair and growth. It is found throughout the body but primarily in muscle. Protein needs can be influenced by diet, the form of exercise undertaken, gender, age, and health status, but a protein intake of 12 to 15 percent of total energy intake is usually sufficient. Higher amounts are thought to be superfluous, even for trained athletes. Protein is not usually a major source of energy, but it is broken down and utilized by the body when carbohydrate and fat stores have been depleted.

FLUID REPLACEMENT

The body loses water all the time but especially during periods of intense exercise. At least 75 percent of the energy expended during exercise is released as heat, and the evaporation of sweat is the primary mechanism for dissipating this heat. Sweat rates vary according to such factors as the intensity of

continued on page 50

Protein building
Exactly how much protein is necessary for top athletic performance is a topic of huge debate. Many bodybuilders and weight lifters believe that a high protein consumption will increase muscle mass and maximize strength. However, it is now thought that a daily intake of just 1.2 to 1.7 grams of protein per kilogram of body weight is sufficient for both speed and strength, as long as enough carbohydrate is consumed. In practice, athletes routinely consume more protein than this and are unlikely to need any extra.

REPLENISHING
Studies involving cyclists show that performance quickly declines if body-fluid and blood-sugar levels drop below normal. Isotonic drinks provide a handy source of both energy and fluid.

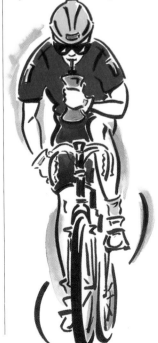

ENERGY-GIVING SPORTS DRINKS

Sport drinks usually contain some sugar and salt, so in addition to replacing fluid and salt lost through sweat, they can provide a rapid source of energy. They come in three types—hypertonic, isotonic, and hypotonic—according to how concentrated the drink is in relation to the blood's own density. Their concentration level determines how quickly the fluid they contain can be absorbed by the body.

HYPERTONIC DRINKS	ISOTONIC DRINKS	HYPOTONIC DRINKS
Have a high carbohydrate content and are denser than the blood, so they are absorbed slowly by the body. Formulated to provide energy rather than replace fluid.	Contain carbohydrates at a level of concentration on a par with those in the blood. Can be drunk before, during, and after exercise, both to replace lost fluid and to provide extra energy.	Contain only a small amount of carbohydrate and are less dense than the blood. Are taken to provide quick fluid replacement rather than for a significant energy boost.

Carbohydrates

One of the most common reasons for failing to complete an exercise session is fatigue. This tiredness is often the result of poor nutrition and a failure to refuel the body with enough carbohydrates and other nutrients.

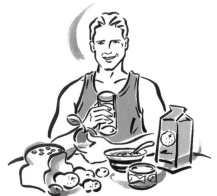

FOOD FOR ACTIVITY

Maintaining a balanced diet that features all the essential food groups in the right proportions is good health advice for everyone. However, if you exercise regularly, you will need greater quantities of certain foods than others. To get the right balance of food for regular exercise, your diet should comprise 55 to 65 percent carbohydrate, 20 to 30 percent fat (mainly from unsaturated forms, such as vegetable and fish oils), and 12 to 15 percent protein, from foods such as lean meat, fish, and legumes. While increasing your carbohydrate consumption is crucial for exercising effectively, you can also regulate the amount and types of other foods you eat—and when you eat them—to get the most benefit from your exercise sessions.

Eating for endurance

Training for endurance, or stamina, places the greatest demands on your body's energy supplies. It is important that you consume enough carbohydrates before, during, and after exercising to fuel these energy needs. Start the day with a good breakfast and eat wholesome snacks throughout the day; you can carry some high-carbohydrate snacks with you. Make use of low-fat products whenever possible. Ideally, avoid adding extra butter or margarine to dishes, cut out fried foods, and eat low-fat or nonfat dairy products and lean meats. You can obtain carbohydrates in liquid form by drinking a glass of fruit juice or a commercial sports drink.

Eating for strength

When exercising to improve your strength, you should still make foods that raise energy levels your priority, not protein, and follow the basic principles of high carbohydrate

EATING FOR EXERCISE

The amount of carbohydrate you need depends upon such factors as weight and level of exercise. Most adults aged 25 to 40 who do moderate exercise each day should include 300 to 400 grams of carbohydrate in their daily diet. The menu below contains 340 to 400 grams of carbohydrate and has enough calories for a moderately active woman who weighs 57 kg (125 pounds).

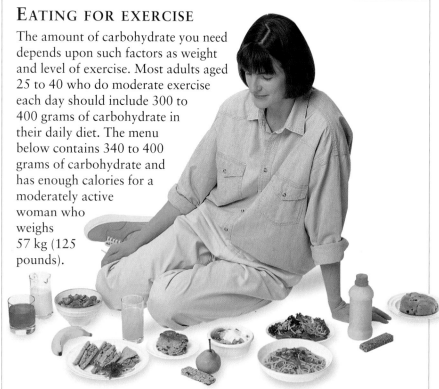

Breakfast (50–70 g)
30 g (1 oz) cereal with 180 ml (6 ounces) skim milk and a few sliced strawberries; 180 ml (6 ounces) fruit juice

Midmorning (15–25 g) 1 banana

Lunch (65–70 g)
Tuna salad and sliced cucumbers on 2 slices of whole-grain bread; 240 ml (8 ounces) mixed vegetable juice

Mid afternoon (30–35 g)
1 pear; 1 snack bar

Dinner (100–105 g)
220 g (8 ounces) cooked spaghetti with Bolognese sauce; mixed greens with olive oil dressing; 170 g (6 ounces) low-fat yogurt or low-fat custard, topped with sliced fruit

Training (30–40 g)
240 ml (8 ounces) fruit juice; 1 snack bar

Evening snack (20–25 g)
180 ml (6 ounces) skim milk; 1 cinnamon bun

intake. If you do not eat sufficient carbohydrate to fuel your energy needs, you will end up using protein as a fuel rather than to build muscle. Protein is essential in your diet, but you should select low-fat sources. Cut visible fat from meat, choose the white meat of poultry more often than red meat, buy canned fish in spring water rather than oil, and choose low-fat or nonfat dairy products rather than whole-milk versions. Legumes are also high in protein and low in fat. Eat a varied diet and combine foods to get the best protein quality—for instance, beans with rice, cereal with milk, peanut butter with whole-grain bread.

Eating for quick energy access

Make sure that your daily diet contains sufficient carbohydrate for all your energy needs. One carbohydrate-loaded meal just prior to training will not compensate for a poor overall diet. If your muscle glycogen levels are likely to be low because of repeated or prolonged periods of exercise, then just prior to an exercise session it is better to eat foods that are low in fiber and have a high glycemic value (see page 46), such as a jam sandwich or a banana. Sports drinks are an easy energy source to take before, during, or after exercise because they are are readily absorbed. (However, if you have high blood pressure, consult your doctor before using a sports drink.)

High energy recipes

The recipes below provide a good intake of carbohydrates to sustain you during exercise, especially if eaten one to two hours before a session.

TAGLIATELLE WITH SHRIMP, ARUGULA, AND TOMATOES

Pasta dishes can be the basis for almost any number of quick, easy-to-make meals that are rich in energy-providing complex carbohydrates.

2 tsp olive oil
1 shallot, finely chopped
1 tbsp chopped parsley
450 g (1 lb) plum tomatoes, peeled, seeded, and chopped

300 ml (1¼ cups) vegetable stock
225 g (8 oz) uncooked shrimp, shelled and deveined
450 g (1 lb) tagliatelle
50 g (2 oz) arugula leaves
Salt and pepper to taste

■In a medium-size saucepan, heat the oil. Add the shallot and cook for 2 to 3 minutes or until soft but not brown.
■Add the parsley, tomatoes, and stock. Bring to a boil, reduce the heat, and simmer for 15 minutes or until thickened. Add the shrimp and cook for 5 minutes.
■Meanwhile, cook the tagliatelle in salted boiling water for 10 to 12 minutes or until al dente. Drain.
■In a warm large serving bowl, toss together the tagliatelle, sauce, and arugula leaves. Add the salt and pepper.
Serves 4

HEARTY VEGETABLE HOTPOT

Root vegetables, such as potatoes, parsnips, turnips, rutabagas, and carrots, make a tasty, carbohydrate-rich casserole.

2 tbsp olive oil
1 large onion, sliced thick
1 stalk celery, sliced
1 kg (2¼ lb) mixed root vegetables, cut into chunks
1 green bell pepper, sliced
2 tbsp all-purpose flour

600 ml (2½ cups) vegetable stock
450 g (1 lb tomatoes), peeled, seeded, and chopped
1 tbsp tomato puree
1 bay leaf
1 sprig thyme
Salt and pepper to taste

■In a large, heavy saucepan, heat the oil. Add the onion and celery and cook for 5 minutes or until soft.
■Add the mixed root vegetables, bell pepper, and flour. Cook, stirring, for 1 minute.
■Add the remaining ingredients and bring the mixture to a boil. Cover and simmer for 25 to 30 minutes or until cooked through. Remove the bay leaf and thyme sprig before serving.
Serves 4

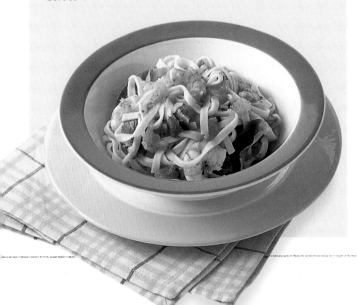

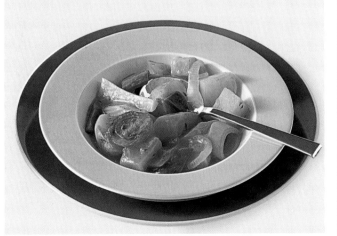

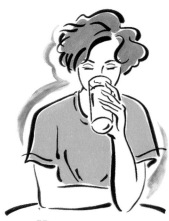

HOMEMADE SPORTS DRINK
You can make your own sports drink, which you can sip during exercise to replace fluid and salt lost through sweat and supply carbohydrates to boost your body's energy stores.

To prepare the drink, add 1 level teaspoon of table salt and up to 8 level teaspoons of sugar to 1 liter (1 quart) of boiling water. Leave the mixture to cool and then store it in the refrigerator in a suitable container until you need it. The sugar content slows the rate at which the water is absorbed. When fluid replacement is the priority, for example on hot and humid days, reduce the level of sugar.

the activity, environmental conditions, and the type of clothing worn. Exercise in hot and humid weather, for example, may result in the loss of up to 2 liters (about 2 quarts) of water per hour. All aerobic activity causes sweating. Even swimmers can lose enough fluid in their sweat to have a detrimental effect on performance; however, because they are in water, swimmers are often unaware of their sweating.

Water must be replaced at regular intervals to prevent dehydration, which can lead to reduced strength, power, and endurance. Even a small loss of fluid can affect performance, while losing more than 4 percent of total body fluid can cause exhaustion and may be dangerous. You should drink a little fluid every 15 to 20 minutes while exercising and up to one liter of fluid before and after an exercise session.

Plain water is the ideal choice for events of less than 60 minutes, since fluid replacement is the main need. However, during periods of intense exertion, particularly in hot weather, the body also loses salt in the sweat, and it must be replaced. Adding a small amount of salt to drinks consumed during and after exercise can be beneficial.

EATING BEFORE EXERCISE
You can enhance your performance before exercise by eating a low-fat, carbohydrate-rich, high-GI food, such as a banana, some cereal, or toast with jam.

It is sensible to leave at least one and preferably two hours between eating a large meal and embarking on a training session because blood is diverted away from the muscles to the stomach for digestion. The exact interval is often dictated by the type of activity undertaken. It may be more detrimental to eat before an activity that involves running and jumping because the intense movement may cause nausea. Experiment with different foods prior to exercise to find out which ones you can eat without causing nausea, stomach pains, or other difficulties.

By referring to the Glycemic Index (page 46), you can plan your carbohydrate intake to help ensure optimum performance. Research shows that low-GI foods eaten before prolonged strenuous exercise, such as an all-day hike, increase endurance. Low-GI foods include such fruits as apples, cherries, and peaches; legumes, such as baked beans and chickpeas; and milk and yogurt.

A good meal to have before a hike might be lentil soup, fresh fruit, and yogurt. During the walk, when a more rapid energy supply is needed, a banana, some raisins, or an energy bar would be a good choice.

REPLENISHING ENERGY AFTER EXERCISE
A good way to replenish energy stores is to eat within two hours after exercise because carbohydrates are converted to glycogen faster than usual during this period. Aim to eat 50 grams or more of carbohydrate (1 cup of split pea soup and a slice of bread equal 57 grams). If you are not hungry after exercise, you may find it easier to consume carbohydrate in liquid form—as two glasses of orange juice, for instance—which will replace lost fluid at the same time.

You should eat carbohydrate-rich meals, snacks, or fluids at regular intervals during the 24 hours following exercise to replenish glycogen in the muscles. The choice of carbohydrate will influence how quickly your body is refueled. For optimal refueling, eat foods with a relatively high GI during the two-hour post-exercise period. Ideal foods are bread, bananas, raisins, and breakfast cereals. After this period you should continue to eat high-carbohydrate foods at regular intervals, but they can be of a lower GI, such as pasta and fruit, because your body is no longer rushing to convert them to glucose.

CARBOHYDRATE LOADING

In the days just before a major competitive event, many top athletes follow a diet plan known as carbohydrate loading to increase their glycogen reserves. Maximum glycogen storage is achieved in the 72 hours prior to an event by reducing training and following a high-carbohydrate diet.

During the first 48 hours, they eat meals and snacks based on complex carbohydrates—bread, pasta, rice, and cereals, for example—avoid fried foods, and keep both fat and protein to a minimum. They also drink plenty of water. During the final 24 hours prior to the event, they consume only simple carbohydrates, such as glucose drinks and fruit juices.

CHAPTER 4

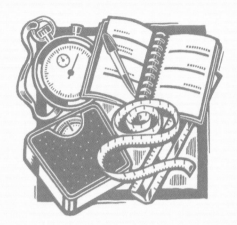

TESTING AND MONITORING

*Before establishing an exercise program,
you should assess your current level of fitness by
measuring your aerobic stamina and your strength,
flexibility, and fat composition. From this starting
point you can then monitor your progress toward
a healthier body and adapt your exercise routine
to match your improved fitness level.*

EVALUATING YOUR FITNESS COMPONENTS

Key indicators of fitness that should be assessed before starting an exercise regimen are stamina (cardiorespiratory endurance), muscular strength, flexibility, and body composition.

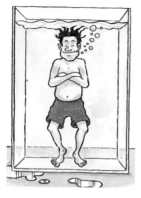

UNDERWATER WEIGHT WATCHERS
Until the 1950s body composition was assessed by determining a subject's weight and the amount of water displaced when he or she was submerged in a tank. Although accurate, this technique was complicated and was eventually abandoned in favor of skin-fold tests.

There are three indicators of overall fitness: stamina, strength, and flexibility. Each of these components needs to be evaluated separately to make a general fitness assessment and pinpoint areas of weakness. For example, one person may have good endurance and muscular strength but poor flexibility; another may be very supple but have limited stamina.

In addition to these three components, many fitness instructors or health clubs will check body composition—height, weight, and percentage of body fat—as part of an overall evaluation of fitness. Besides revealing if there is excess fat, an assessment of body composition can indicate the amount of muscle present and provide markers for improvements that should be made in muscle tone and body shape. These last two are often the reasons people take up exercise in the first place.

Cardiorespiratory fitness, also known as aerobic fitness or stamina, refers to the ability of the heart to pump blood around the body, delivering vital oxygen and nutrients to the muscles. The harder the heart and lungs have to work to meet the body's needs during exercise, the lower the person's level of fitness. Good cardiorespiratory fitness is required to sustain exercise of low to moderate intensity, such as brisk walking or swimming, over relatively long periods. The greater your stamina, the longer you can exercise without tiring.

Muscular strength is the total force that your muscles can exert—for example, the maximum weight you can safely lift—in a single move; muscular endurance is a measure of how many times you can lift that weight. These are important fitness indicators because they reflect your ability to perform everyday tasks, such as carrying

THE SKIN-FOLD TEST

The skin-fold test is the most widely used method of assessing body composition. It is based on the fact that 20 to 70 percent of body fat is found just under the skin, where it is called subcutaneous fat. A device called a calliper (above) is used to measure the thickness of a fold of skin at one of several possible sites on the body, and a mathematical formula is then used to estimate the total amount of body fat, taking into account the person's age and sex.

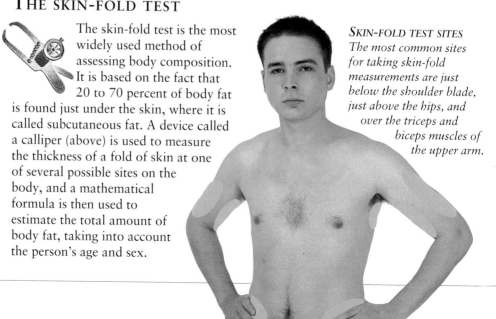

SKIN-FOLD TEST SITES
The most common sites for taking skin-fold measurements are just below the shoulder blade, just above the hips, and over the triceps and biceps muscles of the upper arm.

ARE YOU READY FOR EXERCISE?

The following questionnaire can help you decide whether you should seek medical advice before starting to exercise. If you answer yes to any of the questions below, see your doctor before increasing your activity levels. People aged 70 years or older should always consult a doctor before starting an exercise program.

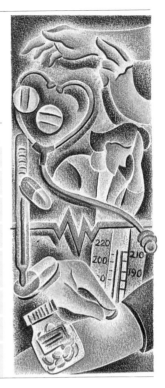

ASK YOURSELF . . .	YES	NO
Has a doctor ever said that you have heart trouble?		
Do you suffer frequently from chest pains?		
Do you often feel faint or have spells of dizziness?		
Have you ever had high blood pressure?		
Has a doctor ever told you that you have a bone or joint problem, such as arthritis, that has been or could be aggravated by exercise?		
Are you age 69 or older and not accustomed to any exercise?		
Are you taking any medication for heart problems or high blood pressure?		
Do you become breathless when walking upstairs?		

shopping bags or lifting bulky items. Many tasks also require the body to twist or stretch in various directions. Although such activity doesn't call for large amounts of strength or stamina, it does demand a degree of all-round flexibility to avoid injury.

ASSESSING YOUR FITNESS

Testing your basic fitness level is important for several reasons. First, it indicates the intensity at which you should begin exercising. (Measuring your heart rate is the easiest way to do this—see page 54.) You will then be able to set yourself reasonable and attainable goals. These are crucial for maintaining motivation and helping you to achieve real improvements in fitness.

Second, identifying your strengths and weaknesses in the various components of fitness will help you to concentrate some of your exercise efforts on areas that are most in need of improvement. For example, if you have good strength but poor flexibility, you may focus on stretching exercises.

The initial testing will also establish a baseline fitness level, so that any change can be monitored in subsequent testing. This will help you see any improvements you have made, which will give you a sense of achievement, and will also allow you to make changes in your program if you find you are not making adequate progress.

ASSESSING YOUR HEALTH

Before starting an exercise program, you should assess your current state of health. Although most people need only to follow basic safety rules when exercising, there are some health conditions, such as arthritis and diabetes, that require special care.

Generally, young and active people who have a low risk of heart disease can start an exercise regimen without seeking medical advice. Older persons who have been inactive for a number of years should be examined by a doctor before beginning an exercise program. It is essential that anyone with symptoms of heart disease, regardless of age, have a medical evaluation before increasing activity levels.

You should avoid exercise if you are suffering the symptoms of an active infection, such as a chesty cough or high temperature. Once you are fully recovered, you can begin with light exercise and build up your activity levels slowly.

If you have been advised to take up exercise for medical reasons—because you are overweight, for instance, or have high blood pressure or high cholesterol—your doctor should be involved in testing your current level of fitness and planning your training schedule. In this way he or she can monitor any improvements that you would not be able to measure yourself.

GET YOUR BLOOD PRESSURE CHECKED
If you suffer unexplained dizziness, breathlessness, or headaches, you may be suffering from high blood pressure, also called hypertension. Before starting a regular fitness program, ask your doctor to give you a full physical checkup that includes a blood-pressure reading.

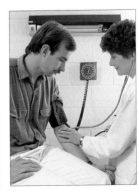

Cardiorespiratory Assessment

You can use the tests featured on these pages to help you measure the efficiency of your cardiorespiratory system. The more oxygen that your heart and lungs can transport to your muscles, the greater your capacity for endurance exercise.

The first step in measuring cardiorespiratory fitness is to determine your resting heart rate by taking your pulse when you are inactive. The lower your heart rate at rest, the more efficiently your heart is working. The next step is to take your pulse 30 seconds after a period of fairly energetic exercise, such as the 3-minute step test (opposite page). This shows how quickly your heart recovers from physical exertion. The lower the heart rate, the fitter you are.

TWO WAYS TO TAKE YOUR PULSE

You can take your pulse at the wrist or neck. Measure your resting pulse in the morning before getting up. It will probably be between 50 and 100 beats per minute (bpm). Take your recovery pulse rate 30 seconds after energetic exercise. Your pulse will be slowing down as you do this, so for accuracy, count the beats for 15 seconds and multiply by 4.

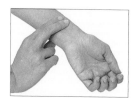

WRIST PULSE
To take your pulse at the wrist, place two fingers just below the base of the thumb.

Make it accurate
Count the pulse beats for 15 seconds and multiply by 4 for an accurate pulse reading.

NECK PULSE
To take a neck pulse, place two fingers halfway between the windpipe and the muscle at the side of the neck.

ASSESSING YOUR PULSE RATES

These charts provide guidelines to help you assess your resting and recovery pulse rates based on your age and gender. If your resting pulse rate is in the poor category, it is inadvisable to assess your own recovery pulse rate. Instead, get a full medical checkup and ask a fitness expert to devise a suitable exercise regimen.

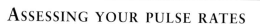

RESTING PULSE RATE				
AGE	POOR	FAIR	GOOD	EXCELLENT
MEN				
20–29	86+	70–84	62–68	60 or less
30–39	86+	72–84	64–70	62 or less
40–49	90+	74–88	66–72	64 or less
50+	90+	76–88	68–74	66 or less
WOMEN				
20–29	96+	78–94	72–76	70 or less
30–39	98+	80–96	72–78	70 or less
40–49	100+	80–98	74–78	72 or less
50+	104+	84–102	76–82	74 or less

RECOVERY PULSE RATE				
AGE	POOR	FAIR	GOOD	EXCELLENT
MEN				
20–29	102+	86–100	76–84	74 or less
30–39	102+	88–100	80–86	78 or less
40–49	106+	90–104	82–88	80 or less
50+	106+	92–104	84–90	82 or less
WOMEN				
20–29	112+	94–110	88–92	86 or less
30–39	114+	96–112	88–94	86 or less
40–49	116+	96–114	90–94	88 or less
50+	118+	100–116	92–98	90 or less

THE 3-MINUTE STEP TEST

In this test you step onto and off a step or sturdy box continuously for exactly 3 minutes and then wait 30 seconds before taking your recovery pulse rate (see opposite page). The lower your heart rate, the fitter you are.

In order to work to the correct pace during the 3-minute session, it can help to use a metronome. Men should aim for 24 complete steps per minute, for which the metronome should be set to 96 beats per minute; women should aim for a rate of 22 complete steps per minute, which equals 88 metronome beats per minute. While it is not essential to use a metronome, you might need to do the test two or three times before you discover the correct pace at which to work. In order to get an accurate assessment of your cardio-respiratory fitness, make sure you allow yourself plenty of time to recover between step tests.

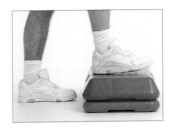

1 *Step up onto the box with the right foot, making sure that the heel touches first, and then follow with the left foot.*

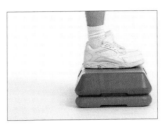

2 *When both feet are flat on the box, transfer your weight to your right foot and step down to the ground with the left foot and then the right.*

ONE STEP AT A TIME
Full weight should be transferred to the leading foot before lifting the other foot onto the step. Keep looking straight ahead.

Keep to the beat
A metronome can help you keep a steady rhythm. Set it to 96 bpm for men and 88 bpm for women. Each step has four beats—up/up/down/down.

THE 1-MILE WALK TEST

This test estimates your level of cardiorespiratory fitness based on the time it takes you to walk exactly 1 mile as fast as you can. It is recommended for people who know they have a low fitness level or who have been inactive for a long period. A reasonably fit person should be able to do it in under 15 minutes. If it takes more than 20 minutes, you are not fit. By doing this test once a month, you will be able to assess how much you have improved.

Up your pace
Cover the distance as fast as possible without becoming too breathless. Aim to raise your heart rate above 120 beats per minute.

WALK TALL
Keep your head up, don't carry anything, and wear light clothes and comfortable shoes. Avoid slouching.

Arms should remain relaxed and swing in time with the opposite leg.

Steps should be the longest you can comfortably manage.

PLANNING YOUR 1-MILE ROUTE

In order to do the walk test, you will need a suitable route. You can choose a stretch of pavement near your home, ideally away from heavy traffic, or find an area of open land, such as a sports field or running track. Before you start, measure 1 mile (about 1,600 meters or 1,760 yards). You can use a map to determine the distance or, if following a road, drive along the route beforehand and use the car's odometer to measure out half a mile. There and back will give you the correct distance. If you are using a club's sports field or track, the officials should be able to tell you its length.

Assessing Strength

Assessing strength is a way of gauging the ability of the muscles to repeat identical movements or to hold a load or position for a period of time. Improving muscle strength will enable you to carry out physical activities longer without tiring.

THE ABDOMINAL CURL TEST

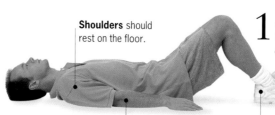

When doing abdominal curls, your feet should not be held in position by anything, because this transfers the effort to the legs rather than the abdominal muscles. You should also keep your arms relaxed at your sides and avoid using them to provide extra leverage. To gauge your standard, compare the total number of curls you complete in 1 minute with the figures in the tables below and keep a record so you can monitor your progress.

Shoulders should rest on the floor.

Arms should be relaxed with palms facing down.

Feet should be flat on the floor and unrestricted.

1 Lie on your back with your knees at 90 degrees and feet flat on the floor. Rest your shoulders on the floor and fully extend your arms by your sides with the palms of the hands facing down.

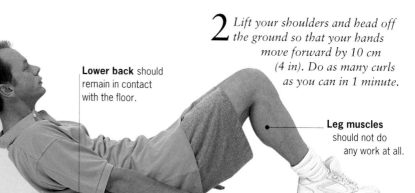

Lower back should remain in contact with the floor.

Leg muscles should not do any work at all.

2 Lift your shoulders and head off the ground so that your hands move forward by 10 cm (4 in). Do as many curls as you can in 1 minute.

Make it controlled
Make sure that you move only your upper back and arms throughout the maneuver. This will ensure that only your abdominal muscles are being used to lift the upper body.

ABDOMINAL CURL TEST—MUSCLE ENDURANCE RATING

The abdominal curl test is widely used as an index of muscle strength and endurance because the abdominal muscles play a crucial role in stabilizing the body and ensuring good posture. Compare your results with the tables below, which show the average ratings for men and women according to age.

MEN					
AGE	VERY LOW	LOW	MODERATE	HIGH	VERY HIGH
29 or under	below 38	38–41	42–47	48–52	52+
30–39	below 30	30–33	34–39	40–44	44+
40–49	below 25	25–28	29–34	35–39	39+
50–59	below 20	20–23	24–29	30–34	34+
60–69	below 15	15–18	19–24	25–29	29+

WOMEN					
AGE	VERY LOW	LOW	MODERATE	HIGH	VERY HIGH
29 or under	below 34	34–37	38–43	44–48	48+
30–39	below 26	26–30	31–35	36–40	40+
40–49	below 21	21–23	24–30	31–35	35+
50–59	below 16	16–19	20–25	26–30	30+
60–69	below 11	11–14	15–20	21–25	25+

Measuring Flexibility

Flexibility is specific for every joint of the body. However, the test most commonly used as a measure of overall flexibility is known as the sit-and-reach test. It indicates the suppleness in the lower back muscles and hamstrings.

THE MODIFIED SIT-AND-REACH TEST

For this test you will need a long ruler, a sturdy box, and a partner to help you. Start by sitting on the floor with your back and head resting against a wall and your legs fully extended with both feet against the box.

Back should be kept straight.

Do not bounce your muscles in order to reach farther.

Measure to your fingertips

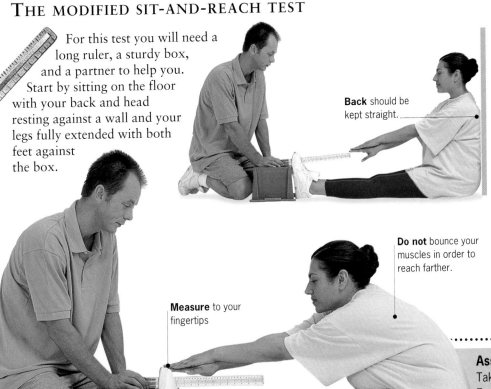

1 *Place one hand on top of the other and reach toward the box without moving your head and back away from the wall. Meanwhile, your partner should rest one end of the ruler on the box and align the other end of it with your fingertips. This is your starting reference point.*

2 *While your partner holds the ruler firmly in place, slowly lean forward, moving your head and shoulders away from the wall, and slide your fingertips as far along the ruler as possible.*

Assess your progress
Take the farthest of three trials. Each time record the distance from your starting point to the end of your range of motion.

MODIFIED SIT-AND-REACH SCORES

The figures below show average sit-and-reach scores (in inches) for men and women according to age (multiply by 2.54 to convert to centimeters). There is no single measure of flexibility; the figures are intended as a general guide only. If you suffer from back or muscle disorders, seek medical advice before taking this test.

MEN					
AGE	VERY LOW	LOW	MODERATE	HIGH	VERY HIGH
35 or under	below 9	9–13	13–15	15–18	18+
36–49	below 8	8–13	11–14	14–16	16+
50+	below 8	8–9	9–12	12–15	15+

WOMEN					
AGE	VERY LOW	LOW	MODERATE	HIGH	VERY HIGH
35 or under	below 10	10–15	15–16	16–18	18+
36–49	below 10	10–12	12–15	15–18	18+
50+	below 8	8–9	9–12	12–15	15+

Assessing Body Composition

Measuring your body composition will tell you how much fat you have relative to your muscle. The lower the ratio of fat you have, the fitter you are likely to be and the less risk you will have of contracting such disorders as heart disease.

In the past changes in body composition were assessed using weight and height tables that gave a standard weight range for a given height. These tables were often misleading. For example, a man who has done a lot of weight training will have put on muscle and gained weight. This does not mean that he is obese but that he has a greater ratio of lean body weight to fat tissue. More accurate ways to assess changes in body composition are now used, namely, the waist-to-hip ratio and the body mass index (BMI).

BODY MASS INDEX

To determine your BMI, weigh yourself in kilograms, wearing minimal clothing. (To convert pounds to kilograms, divide by 2.2.) Then measure your height in meters from the top of your scalp. (To convert inches to meters, divide by 39.37.) Multiply your height by itself and divide this figure into your weight to determine your BMI. For example, if you are 1.7 m tall and weigh 65 kg, multiply 1.7 by 1.7, then divide 65 by 2.89—your BMI is 22.5. Being overweight is defined as having a BMI of more than 25. A BMI above 30 is associated with health risks like heart disease, stroke, and diabetes.

BMI scale
The table below shows the average range of BMI readings for the general population.

AGE GROUP (YEARS)	BMI
19–24	19–24
25–34	20–25
35–44	21–26
45–54	22–27
55–65	23–28
over 65	24–29

WAIST-TO-HIP RATIO

The waist-to-hip ratio is a way of comparing the amount of fat deposited in the upper body (waist) with that in the lower body (hips). To find your ratio, divide your hip measurement by your waist measurement. A healthy waist-to-hip ratio is 1.0 or lower in men and 0.85 or lower in women. The places where fat is most likely to be deposited often vary between men and women. Women have a tendency to store fat in their breasts, arms, and thighs, whereas men predominantly deposit fat on their waist and abdomen. Research indicates that the waist-to-hip ratio is a good predictor of future health because too much fat in the abdominal area seems to be associated with such medical problems as heart disease and certain forms of cancer.

Measuring waist and hips
Measure your waist just above the top of your hip bones, where your body naturally curves in. Measure your hips at their widest point.

ACHIEVING YOUR FITNESS GOALS

To get the most from your exercise program, it is important to set yourself clear fitness goals, gain an understanding of the principles of exercise, and maintain your motivation.

Once you have assessed your current level of fitness, you can use the information to identify the areas that most need attention. Your priority might be to raise your cardiorespiratory fitness or to improve flexibility or strength.

It is important to continue assessing your fitness at regular intervals. Repeated assessment will indicate whether your fitness is improving at an adequate rate. If it is not, you might decide to revise your exercise schedule—perhaps by increasing the intensity or amount of exercise or by changing the type of activity—in order to reach some of your fitness goals sooner.

Take some time to think about the reasons you want to become more active. You may want or need to lose weight or have a desire to feel generally healthier; or your goal might be something more concrete, like getting fit to go on vacation or to take part in a marathon. Even if your reasons are very general in nature, they will still help to keep you going. In addition, the desired results will form a basis from which you can set specific goals.

SETTING GOALS

To stay motivated, it can help to set yourself short-term, easily attainable goals, as well as more demanding long-term ones. Each time you achieve one of these goals, your morale will be boosted, encouraging you in the drive toward a fitter, healthier body.

Your goals should be challenging but realistic. They must also be easily achievable because the failure to reach them could lead not only to disappointment but also to abandonment of the program. For example, if it currently takes you 20 minutes to walk a mile (1.6 kilometers), it would be more realistic

to set a starting target of 19 rather than 15 minutes. You should also try to be as specific as possible in your chosen targets, as this will give your program more focus. For instance, rather than setting yourself the global aim of increasing your overall muscle strength, you might set a target of increasing the number of push-ups you can perform from 5 to 10, then from 10 to 15.

Some of your goals should also be short-term so you can reach them within a time frame that keeps you motivated. For example, in addition to setting yourself the goal of losing 11 kilograms (25 pounds) in total, you could aim to lose 1.3 kilograms (3 pounds) per month. By setting yourself a series of such targets, you're more likely to achieve success in the short term and go on to satisfy your ultimate aims.

EXERCISE ACHIEVERS

Some extraordinary exercise goals have been achieved by people determined to succeed. In 1993 a 60-year-old Venezuelan violin maker became the oldest person to climb Mount Everest. Another remarkable milestone was reached by Madge Sharples, who proved it is never too late to start a fitness regimen. Mrs. Sharples did no exercise at all until the age of 62, when she started practicing yoga. She went on to include sessions of swimming, body building, and weight lifting in her exercise routine. She ran her first marathon at the age of 64 and only gave up running in the London Marathon at the age of 73.

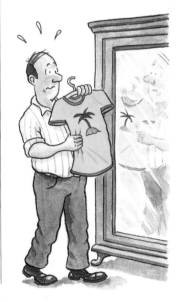

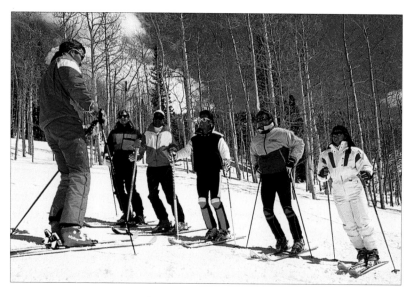

too much may do more harm than good by putting excess strain on muscles and joints before they have had time to adapt.

The amount of exercise that your body must perform in order to produce the desired effect depends on several factors. These include your current level of fitness, your specific exercise goals, and the various components of fitness that you want to improve. It is also important to remember that you will have to continue to push yourself; once your strength or fitness has improved to the point that your current level of exercise is too easy, for example, you will need to increase your output in order to achieve any effect.

To help you decide how to raise your level of exercise at a steady rate, you should bear in mind five principal factors—frequency, intensity, time, type, and maintenance.

Frequency

Improving your fitness requires regular exercise, although the frequency required will depend on the fitness component being worked on and your current and desired condition. Generally speaking, you will have to exercise three to five times a week to promote any changes in your level of fit-

LOOKING FORWARD
An exercise program that is geared toward a clearly definable goal, such as getting fit for a skiing vacation, will give you extra incentive to keep going, even when you are feeling a little under par.

PRINCIPLES OF TRAINING

Your cardiorespiratory system and muscle groups will improve in fitness only if they have to work harder than they usually do. In other words, you have to push your body's physical limits in order to improve your condition; otherwise, you will just remain at the same level. This is called overload adaptation, and it is important that you find the right balance. Too little overload will produce no effect at all, whereas

---

FITNESS DIARY

A detailed fitness diary can provide a useful source of information to monitor and assess your fitness levels and to help you set out new goals and objectives.

As a record of achievement, it will allow you to chart your progress and help boost your motivation to keep striving for improvement.

Set fitness goals
every two weeks and plan each session to help you achieve them.

KEEP IT SHORT
By limiting the fitness program to two weeks at a time, you will find it easier to focus on your goals.

Fitness Goals
Improve time to walk 2 miles.
Increase number of skips.

Exercise Sessions—Week 1
☐ 1 min. abdominal curls _____ (no.)
☐ 2-mile walk _____ (time)
☐ 20-min. swim _____ (no. lengths)
☐ 3-min. jump rope _____ (no.)
☐ 5-mile cycle _____ (time)

Ratings
Resting pulse rate: _____ (bpm)
Recovery pulse rate: _____ (bpm)

Comments
Abdominals were sore after curls.
I was out of breath after jumping rope.

Fitness Goals
Improve number of abdominal curls.
Swim more lengths in 20 minutes.

Exercise Sessions—Week 2
☐ 1 min. abdominal curls _____ (no.)
☐ 2-mile walk _____ (time)
☐ 20-min. swim _____ (no. lengths)
☐ 3-min. jump rope _____ (no.)
☐ 5-mile cycle _____ (time)

Ratings
Resting pulse rate: _____ (bpm)
Recovery pulse rate: _____ (bpm)

Comments
Abdominals were less sore after curls.
I swam 1 more length than last week.

As you complete
each session, check it off so that you can see each training period as a mini goal and its completion as an achievement in itself.

A HEALTHY HEART

For exercise that achieves real aerobic benefits, you must make your heart work harder than it normally does while still staying within safe limits. When you start your fitness regimen, you should aim to exercise at an intensity that pushes your heart rate to 65 percent of its maximum capacity and increase the intensity as you improve. To avoid ill effects, however, never push your heart to more than 85 percent of maximum output. Maximum heart rate is 220 minus your age; for a healthy 50-year-old this would be 170 beats per minute. Therefore, the target heart rate zone for training would be between 111 bpm (170×0.65) and 145 bpm (170×0.85).

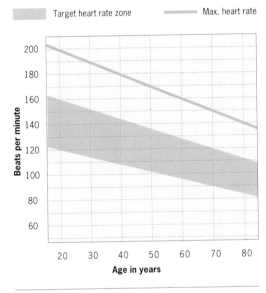

Target heart rate zone ——— Max. heart rate

(Graph: Beats per minute vs. Age in years)

ness. Once you have achieved the desired level, two or three sessions a week may be sufficient to maintain it.

Intensity

Intensity of exercise must be greater than that normally experienced to produce a change. To improve cardiorespiratory fitness, most people exercise at between 65 and 85 percent of maximum heart rate (see above). To check whether you are working at the correct intensity, take your pulse at regular intervals as you exercise. Start at the bottom of the range and work up.

Alternatively, you can use your body's response to exertion to gauge the intensity of the exercise (see page 36). As your fitness program progresses, you will be able to gauge the intensity. You should aim to do some exercise at about level three on the five-point scale (somewhat breathless but can still talk). As you grow fitter and your body adapts, you will find that you perceive the exercise as being easier, in which case you may grade the intensity as level two. When this happens, it is time to increase the intensity so that once again you perceive the effort as being around level three.

Time

To improve cardiorespiratory fitness, it is usually necessary to exercise for a minimum of 20 minutes three times a week and to increase the time as you become fitter. However, the duration of the activity is largely dependent upon the intensity of the exercise. The more intense a particular exercise session, the less time you will be able to spend doing it. For example, you can't sprint for as long as you can jog.

Type

When considering what form of exercise you are going to use to improve your fitness, you should first take into account any specific health needs. For example, if you suffer from osteoporosis, you might consider including such weight-bearing activities as walking and running. However, always seek your doctor's advice first if you have a medical condition that might be affected by exercise. The other critical aspect is to choose an exercise that you enjoy. If you do not find it stimulating, you risk boredom or lack of motivation.

Once you have chosen an exercise that holds your interest, vary your program regularly. Don't let the routine become boring. If you don't want to change the type of exercise, then change the place where you do it—try a new run or cycle route or different people to exercise with. Changes like these will help maintain your interest.

Maintenance

The final principle of exercise is that you must aim to maintain your level of fitness. Any gain is quickly lost if you return to a previously inactive lifestyle. This loss in fitness is very rapid; perhaps as much as half the gains that have been made overall can be lost in as little as two weeks. The simple message is to use it or lose it.

Maintaining your motivation

Exercising for its own sake can be a chore that becomes increasingly difficult to keep up. To stay motivated, look for ways to make exercise enjoyable and interesting. Besides choosing activities that you really like, you can encourage a friend to take up exercise so that you can give each other encouragement. Also, vary your activities or try to find attractive new places for working out to avoid becoming bored.

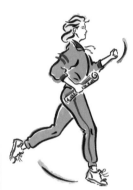

EXTRA EXERCISE
Incorporate more exercise into your everyday tasks, such as jogging to the store for a morning newspaper.

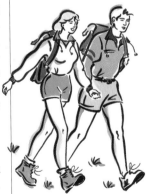

TWO IS COMPANY
Exercise with a friend; you can provide support for each other and make the exercise sessions more fun.

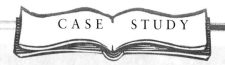

A Misguided Exerciser

Regular aerobic exercise is vital for physical and emotional health. Optimum health, however, comes from following a fitness regimen that includes a variety of activities so that all the muscle groups get a thorough workout. It is also important not to underestimate the importance of other lifestyle factors, such as diet and stress.

Wendy is a 38-year-old marketing manager in a large firm. Her job involves long and often irregular hours, which can be very stressful, but the situation is made worse by the fact that she finds it difficult to delegate. Her husband, Tony, is a maintenance engineer, and his job is stressful at times too.

Despite the fact that they both have demanding careers, Wendy finds that she is expected to cook a meal when she comes home in the evening and to fit laundry and all the other household chores into the week without help from Tony. Wendy also feels that Tony doesn't spend as much time with her as she would like, preferring to socialize with his friends at a bar. He says it's his way of dealing with the stress of his job.

Wendy likes to go for long bicycle rides in the countryside when she wants to unwind. She feels that these cycling sessions provide all the exercise she needs to stay fit.

She is conscious of her figure and limits the calories in her meals in order to keep her weight down. Unfortunately, she finds she gets very tired, especially when doing the housework, and her legs ache after she has been on the go all day. She has also developed a nagging pain in her lower back, which is getting worse. She has had to stop cycling at the moment because it seems to aggravate the problem.

An extra worry is that her mother suffers from osteoporosis. Wendy wants to do everything that she can to prevent the same thing from happening to her.

The combination of health concerns and work pressures is affecting Wendy's relationship with her husband, and they are having frequent arguments.

EMOTIONAL HEALTH
Physical exercise is a good way of dealing with stress in the short term, but unless underlying problems are addressed, it cannot provide a long-term solution.

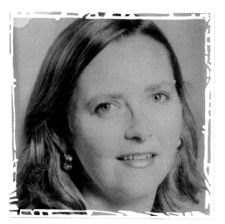

EXERCISE
Activities, such as cycling, that involve only a limited number of muscles in the body do not necessarily provide all-round fitness benefits.

DIET
Even when a diet is low in fat and contains plenty of fruits and vegetables, it is not balanced if it does not provide sufficient energy for your needs.

WORK AND HOME
Combining a busy career with domestic chores can strain a relationship, especially if one partner believes the workload is not being shared equally.

HEALTH
A lifestyle that does not include regular weight-bearing exercise can increase the risk of developing osteoporosis later in life.

WHAT SHOULD WENDY DO?

Wendy went to her doctor for a complete physical examination and learned that there was no underlying medical problem causing the tiredness and back pain. In certain respects Wendy was very healthy, because her heart rate and blood pressure were quite low.

The doctor recommended that Wendy continue to avoid cycling and suggested a program of exercises that would relieve her back pain and strengthen her bones. The doctor advised Wendy to consider joining a health club, where she would get advice on planning a comprehensive exercise routine.

Wendy's doctor also suggested that she take a close look at her diet to make sure it was providing sufficient calories throughout the day, as this might be contributing to her fatigue.

The doctor recommended that Wendy try to delegate more work, both in the office and at home, and set aside some time to sit down with Tony and talk over her grievances. If they could not resolve their difficulties, the doctor suggested that they consider seeking the advice of a marriage counselor.

Wendy and her husband could consider employing someone part-time to do some of the household chores and lighten the load. She might even try to get Tony interested in joining her exercise program.

Action Plan

EMOTIONAL HEALTH
Tackling stress involves a range of measures, not just exercise. Wendy should look at her routine to see if she can manage her time better or share the workload, and rethink priorities so that she is not wasting time on unimportant matters.

EXERCISE
Seek advice on putting together a fitness program that provides an all-over workout but has been specifically tailored to individual needs and lifestyle.

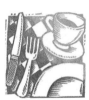

DIET
Don't skip meals, especially breakfast, and make sure all meals have sufficient protein and complex carbohydrates. Consider eating a high-energy snack before an exercise session, when she will be burning up extra calories.

WORK AND HOME
Make sure there is a fair division of labor at home and work and avoid letting resentments build up by failing to air grievances. The first step toward dealing with a relationship problem is for both partners to talk it through.

HEALTH
Exercise like walking, jogging, and aerobic dancing, combined with a diet that includes plenty of calcium, can help build up bone mass and lower the risk of developing osteoporosis later in life.

HOW THINGS TURNED OUT FOR WENDY

Wendy stopped cycling for a while and started going for long walks instead, which she found to be equally good at helping her unwind. She forced herself to delegate more of her office work, and this gave her time to go swimming at lunchtime.

The fitness trainer at Wendy's health club devised a program of aerobic step routines plus muscle-toning and strengthening exercises to strengthen her bones and build up all-around fitness levels. The health club also gave Wendy a diet plan to follow; this included recipes that would put more complex carbohydrates and low-fat protein, such as lean meat and chicken breast, into her diet, as well as suggestions for some high-energy snacks to eat between meals.

Wendy's back pain has greatly eased, and all the exercise she has been doing has given her a healthy appetite without leading to an increase in weight. She now feels far less stressed than before.

Wendy had a heart-to-heart with Tony. He wasn't keen to take on much housework himself, but he did think it was a good idea to employ a housekeeper. Although Tony has not been persuaded to take part in Wendy's fitness sessions at the health club, he does join her on long country walks, which give them time to have heart-to-heart talks.

BEATING THE EXERCISE BLUES

Some people become disheartened by apparent lack of progress, especially in the first few weeks of an exercise regimen. If you feel you are losing momentum, try the following suggestions to help sustain your desire to keep fit.

▶ *Make a list of your goals and reasons for wanting to exercise. See if these goals have changed since you began your routine and make a note of any progress you have made.*

▶ *Try on various garments and see if clothes that fit you before you started exercising are now loose or if clothes that were too tight are now easier to put on.*

▶ *Reassess your regime; try to home in on the areas in which you feel you are making the least progress and then concentrate on these.*

CHANGES YOU CAN EXPECT TO NOTICE

During the early weeks of an exercise program, you will probably not detect much change in your appearance or notice any major physiological adaptation to the increased demands you are placing on your body. However, even after the first few sessions you should feel that the exercise is slightly easier than when you first started. This change in perception probably happens because the interaction between muscle and nervous system adapts quickly to exercise. In essence, the coordination between nerve and muscle becomes more efficient.

4 to 6 weeks

Between weeks 4 and 6 of your routine—depending on the components of fitness you are working on—you should start to see some evidence of changes in the structure of your body. Your clothes should be looser, particularly around the waist. In addition, the muscles that you are exercising predominantly should start to become firmer or more defined. These cosmetic changes will continue as you progress with your prescribed regimen.

8 to 12 weeks

After 8 to 12 weeks of your fitness program, you should notice that you are able to perform much more intense exercise than at the beginning but that subjectively it feels no harder than when you first started exercising. This is a result of cardiorespiratory and muscular changes. At this stage you should be able to detect the cardiorespiratory improvements by measuring your resting heart rate. When compared with the figure recorded before the start of the program, the rate should have decreased, indicating that your heart is stronger and more efficient and needs to beat less often.

You should also notice that you sweat more during exercise than you used to. This is a normal adaptation as the thermostat of the body becomes more efficient and is able to disperse heat produced by the exercise more rapidly.

12 weeks and beyond

At this stage you should be noticing both physical and psychological benefits. You may feel less fatigued by everyday events and be better able to cope with stressful situations. The quality of your sleep will have improved and you will feel healthier. In addition, you will actually feel slightly depressed if you miss an exercise session, owing to the absence of the body's natural mood enhancers, endorphins, which are produced during exercise. Your body will have started anticipating their release, and if this does not occur, you may experience a slight withdrawal sensation.

Origins

The modern Olympic games were founded in 1892 by a Frenchman, Baron Pierre de Coubertin (1863–1937). De Coubertin was an expert in physical fitness, and it was during a study tour of Europe that he conceived the idea of reviving the Olympic games and recapturing the spirit of ancient Greece. He proposed the idea of the games during a lecture at the Sorbonne in Paris in 1892. The first modern Olympic games were held in Athens, Greece, in 1896, approximately 1,500 years after they had last been held.

De Coubertin was an idealist who believed in the original ideals of the ancient Greek Olympics. His maxim was that the most important part of sport was not to win but to take part. It was de Coubertin who declared that Olympic athletes should retain their amateur status in order to promote sportsmanship and excellence for their own sake.

OLYMPIC REBIRTH
In 1894 de Coubertin met representatives of 12 countries, and the International Olympic Committee (IOC) was inaugurated.

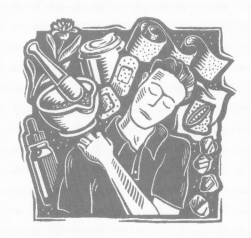

CHAPTER 5

EXERCISING SAFELY

Most injuries suffered during a workout are the result of overexertion or inadequate preparation. By warming up and cooling down before and after exercise, wearing appropriate clothing and footwear, training in moderation, and using good techniques, you can exercise with confidence, knowing that you are working both safely and effectively.

WHEN EXERCISE IS HARMFUL

Although most people can safely take part in a fitness program anytime, there are circumstances under which exercise should be moderated or avoided altogether.

It is now accepted that the risks to health of being inactive far outweigh the risks of being active. But there are some risks associated with exercise, and there are times when extra caution or even abstention from exercise may be necessary. Factors such as illness or pregnancy may require you to rest or make a change in your normal regimen.

ILLNESS AND EXERCISE

Exercising when ill can be dangerous. In the case of minor infections, such as a sore throat, tonsillitis, or earache, gentle exercise is possible when the infection or fever has passed. With active infections, however, especially if there is a fever or muscular aches and pains, exercise should be avoided. A viral infection can cause inflammation of the lymph nodes, lungs, muscles, and heart. Myocarditis (inflammation of the heart muscle) is common to many viral illnesses, including flu and glandular fever, and can be fatal if exercise imposes additional stress.

When the body is fighting an infection, the extra demands of exercise may lower the body's resistance and increase the severity and complications of the illness. Exercise also promotes sweating, which can lead to increased dehydration if you have experienced diarrhea. In addition, exercise may prolong convalescence and increase the risk of depression. After recovering from an illness, you should return to exercise gradually.

Taking medication can cause problems too. Exercise can actually alter the effect of some drugs, as well as increase oxygen consumption and carbon dioxide production. As a consequence you may have to reduce the amount of exercise you do while taking certain medications. If you have any doubts, seek medical advice.

AFTER SURGERY

Most people notice a decline in aerobic fitness and increased feelings of fatigue for at least the first month after major surgery. The deterioration in fitness is similar for both sedentary people and regular exercisers and is proportional to the amount of time spent recovering in bed.

These postoperative changes may be due in part to hormonal responses to surgery, which can affect metabolism and cause temporary immobilization. The extent of the surgery; the loss of muscle mass, body weight, and strength; and reduced aerobic fitness all exacerbate the feelings of fatigue.

Gentle exercise after surgery can offset the damaging physiological effects and speed recovery, enabling you to return to normal activities more quickly. Exercise rehabilitation is now incorporated into the standard care of patients with coronary heart disease, and many doctors advise exercise as soon as possible after discharge from the hospital. Exercise should be of low intensity, build up slowly over a period of months, and be undertaken only on a doctor's advice and after an adequate period of convalescence.

PREGNANCY

Keeping fit helps the body cope with the physical and emotional demands of pregnancy. Regular exercise will not only strengthen the heart and lungs but also help alleviate back pain, aid in weight control, relieve stress, and regulate or prevent gestational diabetes during pregnancy.

Check with your doctor before planning a fitness program. The doctor will take your general health and current fitness level into account. Fatigue and nausea may necessitate a change in routine, and lax ligaments (a

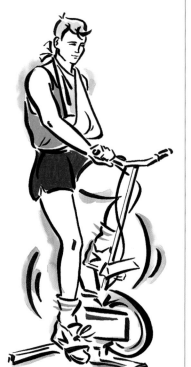

KEEP ACTIVE
Injuries do not have to stop you completely from exercising. Whenever possible, you should try to adapt your training program to compensate for an injury so that you can remain active.

common consequence of pregnancy) may increase the risk of injury. Aerobic exercise should be regular—three to five sessions per week—but last no more than 30 minutes per session. The intensity should be geared toward maintaining optimum health rather than peak performance.

For women who have not exercised regularly before their pregnancy, low-intensity exercise, such as walking, swimming, and stationary cycling, is the most suitable.

After pregnancy

Many of the changes in a woman's body during pregnancy last for weeks or months after the birth, so the return to a full fitness regimen should be gradual. If the delivery was problem-free, exercise can be resumed four to six weeks after the birth or after bleeding has stopped. If the birth involved any complications or surgery, a doctor should be consulted before resuming exercise. Some light strength work will help restore muscle tone and posture, and exercises to strengthen the pelvic floor muscles will help prevent stress incontinence.

Many women suffer lower back or leg pain during pregnancy because of changes in weight and posture. This may continue for a while after the birth, partly because of the hormone relaxin, which continues to cause lax ligaments for several months afterward. Retraining your posture and lifting correctly are vitally important. You

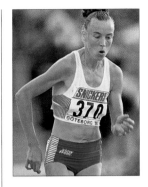

RECORD-BREAKING RECOVERY
Many top women athletes have returned to their sport after giving birth, feeling stronger, fitter, and as dedicated as ever. A few months after becoming a mother, runner Liz McColgan set a new 10,000-meter world record.

PREGNANCY AND EXERCISE

Drink plenty of fluids before, during, and after exercise to keep you and your baby fully hydrated. Maintain a moderate pace and avoid jarring or jumping motions because ligaments are more susceptible to injury during pregnancy. Wear properly fitted training shoes and keep your stretches slow and gentle.

HEAD AND NECK
To relieve tension in your head, neck, and shoulders, gently tilt your head to one side and then straighten it. Repeat to the other side. Perform this movement twice to each side.

Keep your back straight and your arms relaxed.

ARMS AND SHOULDERS
To ease aching arms, raise one arm above your head and bend it at the elbow. Grasp your elbow with the other hand and gently pull toward your head to feel the stretch.

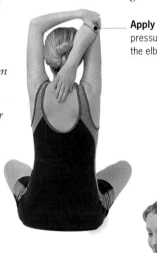

Apply gentle pressure to the elbow.

Feel the stretch through your spine.

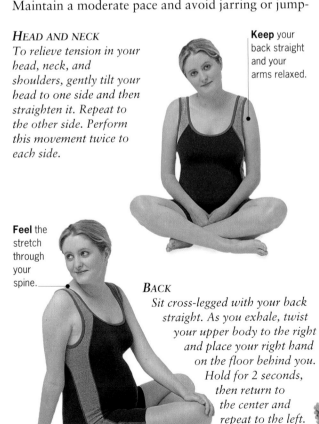

BACK
Sit cross-legged with your back straight. As you exhale, twist your upper body to the right and place your right hand on the floor behind you. Hold for 2 seconds, then return to the center and repeat to the left.

LEGS AND FEET
Sit with your back straight and your legs straight in front of you. Place your hands on the floor beside your hips and slowly bend and straighten each knee in turn. Then draw small circles in the air with each foot. Repeat 3 times.

Iron discipline

Women need 10 to 15 mg of dietary iron a day during their reproductive years (twice as much during pregnancy); their training diet should contain such iron-rich foods as fortified cereals, seafood, spinach, and dried fruits. Standard servings are given below.

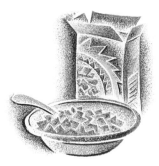

30 g (1 oz) fortified bran cereal contains 10 mg of iron.

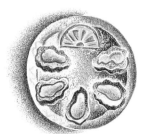

Six medium oysters contain 16.5 mg of iron.

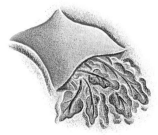

142 g (5 oz) spinach, cooked, contains 4.4 mg iron.

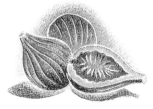

Five dried figs contain 2 mg of iron.

should continue flexibility exercises but avoid stretching to the limits of your range of motion. After pregnancy it takes some time for the abdominal muscles to return to normal, and overworking them can cause permanent damage. It is better not to do standard abdominal curls and sit-ups from lying flat during the first three months.

Wearing a well-fitted support bra when exercising is important because breasts are heavier during pregnancy and nursing, and supporting ligaments are easily stretched. Women who are breast-feeding should feed the baby before exercise and limit any weight loss to no more than 0.5 kilograms (1 pound) a week. In addition to well-balanced meals, they should eat nutritious snacks and drink plenty of water.

OVEREXERCISING

Overexercising is a problem associated more commonly with competitive athletes than with the average exerciser, but it is easy to push yourself beyond safe levels. Common signs of overexercising include impaired immunity, iron deficiency anemia, susceptibility to injury, excessive weight loss, and menstrual disorders.

Impaired immunity

While moderate exercise is believed to boost the immune system, there is evidence that strenuous exercise can harm it. For reasons not fully understood, the immune system appears to be suppressed by overtraining, and people who regularly engage in very strenuous exercise may be more prone to illness and infection. Indeed, athletes seem to have an unusually high incidence of upper respiratory infections. A study of marathon runners in the United States found a two-fold increase in respiratory infections among athletes who ran more than 100 kilometers (about 60 miles) a week.

Iron deficiency anemia

Iron is a vital component of the pigment hemoglobin in red blood cells and is the principal means of transporting oxygen in the blood. Iron deficiency leads to reduced levels of hemoglobin, a condition known as anemia, which causes general sluggishness, fatigue, and loss of appetite. Excessive exercise is thought to promote a high degree of iron loss through the destruction of red blood cells. Women are more susceptible to

> **CAUTION**
> *Anyone who suspects an iron deficiency should have a blood test to confirm it and take supplements only under the supervision of a nutritionist or doctor. Too much iron can lead to iron overload, which can damage the heart.*

anemia, owing to the extra loss of iron through menstrual bleeding, and pregnant women who exercise strenuously face an even greater drain on their iron stores because of the demands of the baby.

Susceptibility to injury

Continuous, excessive exercise can cause muscle pain and tissue damage that in time may progress to more serious problems, including muscle tears and stress fractures. To avoid injury, reduce your level of exercise as soon as you feel any discomfort.

Excessive weight loss

Intensive training can often lead to weight loss, sometimes because it causes a loss of appetite but more often as a result of energy expenditure exceeding energy intake. If the weight loss is rapid, progressive muscle wasting, loss of body fat, and a low blood-sugar level may result. Because productive muscle mass is lost, performance and the ability to sustain exercise are likely to be impaired. Extreme weight loss in women may lead to further complications, such as menstrual disorders.

Menstrual disorders

Menstrual problems, such as irregular periods (oligomenorrhea) and the cessation of periods (amenorrhea), are more common among women who do strenuous exercise. Intensive exercise can also lead to delayed menarche (onset of menstruation). The disruption to the menstrual cycle may be associated with low levels of body fat or extreme weight loss, hormonal fluctuations resulting from sustained intense exercise, or the psychological stress associated with intensive training. While there appears to be no lasting or irreversible effects on the reproductive system, there is concern that athletes who experience menstrual disorders may be at greater risk of developing osteoporosis.

PREPARING FOR EXERCISE

Good preparation reduces the risk of injury during exercise. Choose suitable clothing and footwear and have a warm-up before each exercise session and a cool-down afterward.

The correct clothing to wear during exercise depends on the activity you are undertaking and the conditions under which you are doing it. If you are in a gym doing a moderate to intense workout, for example, lightweight clothing will prevent you from overheating. If you are running outside in the cold, several layers of warm clothing are preferable.

Similarly, it is crucial that you choose the correct footwear for different activities because many injuries result from wearing the wrong type of training shoes. Running shoes, for instance, should not be worn for an aerobics class because they provide little support for the ankles, which could result in a sprain or other joint damage.

CLOTHING

Because it is absorbent, cool, and comfortable against the skin, clothing made of cotton is preferred by many people for exercise. Certain synthetic clothes that are touted as having the ability to wick away perspiration may actually be more comfortable in certain circumstances because they allow perspiration to evaporate rather than absorb into the material. Whichever material you prefer, any style you select should be nonbinding.

Being visible is an important consideration for anyone who exercises on roads or pathways, especially in the early morning or at night. If you cycle, run, or jog, it is essential to wear bright clothing and reflective bibs and/or armbands.

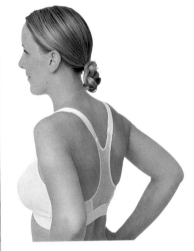

VITAL SUPPORT
Wearing a sports bra when exercising is a good idea, not only for comfort but also for the long-term protection of the suspensory ligaments that support the breasts.

THE SPORTS WARDROBE

Clothing should be comfortable and should not restrict movement. To prevent overheating, material that comes into contact with the skin should be porous, allowing perspiration to evaporate and letting air in to cool the body.

THE IMPORTANCE OF LAYERING
Wearing layers makes it easier to control your temperature by removing or adding items of clothing.

Inner layers

Outer layers

Middle layers

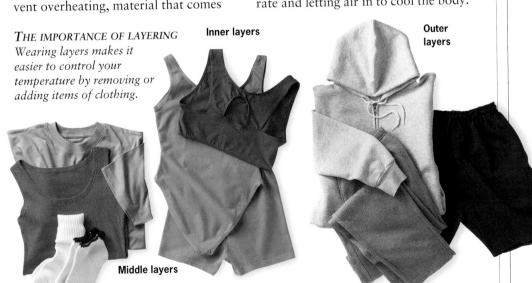

Prevent Injury

Warming up and cooling down are vital components of any exercise program. Too often, however, they are either carried out inadequately or are overlooked altogether, and often the result is unnecessary pain and injury.

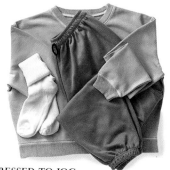

DRESSED TO JOG
Wearing a sweat suit in cool weather helps prevent injury by keeping the muscles and joints warm.

The extent to which you need to warm up and cool down depends on the intensity and duration of your fitness session, environmental factors like temperature and humidity, and your physical condition. Follow these guidelines on how to warm up effectively before your exercise session and cool down thoroughly afterward to ensure that you exercise at your optimum level and reduce the risk of injury.

WARM-UP ROUTINE

Your warm-up should last 8 to 10 minutes and include exercises to aid mobility and raise your pulse. Mobility exercises—which include shoulder circles, arm circles, knee lifts, and hip circles—are free and easy and move your joints in a controlled manner, helping to warm and circulate the synovial fluid. Pulse-raising activities include brisk walking, gentle jogging, and jumping jacks to gradually raise your pulse and prepare the cardiovascular system. During this part of the warm-up, you should feel warm and breathe more rapidly than normal.

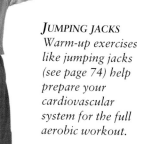

JUMPING JACKS
Warm-up exercises like jumping jacks (see page 74) help prepare your cardiovascular system for the full aerobic workout.

Static warm-up stretching
Warm-up stretches help prepare the muscle fibers to be lengthened safely. Stretches should be static (held still), maintained for 6 to 10 seconds each, and performed only when your muscles are already warm—after the pulse-raising activities. Most exercises involve the major leg muscles, including the calves, hamstrings, and quads, so always include stretches for these in the routine.

COOLING-DOWN PROCEDURE

A cool-down should last for at least 5 minutes and include both pulse-reducing exercises and stretches. As their name suggests, pulse-reducing exercises gradually return your cardiovascular system to its pre-exercise state. You can use the same exercises as in the pulse-raising section of the warm–up. For the cool-down, however, gradually reduce the speed and intensity of the exercise so that, for example, you slow from a jog to a walk, to let your muscles cool slowly.

Static cool-down stretching
Your cool-down is an ideal time to improve flexibility because the muscles are already thoroughly warmed. It is most effective to do cool-down stretches in comfortable positions on the floor or on a mat. Hold stretches longer than during your warm-up: 10 to 30 seconds or more. When stretching, try to relax, ease slowly into the stretches, and hold them still. As you stretch, you should feel mild tension in the bulky part of the muscle but no pain.

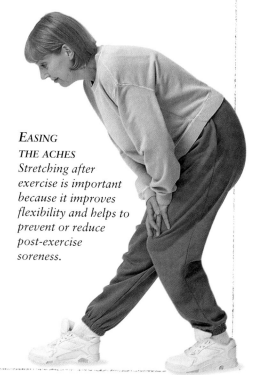

EASING THE ACHES
Stretching after exercise is important because it improves flexibility and helps to prevent or reduce post-exercise soreness.

FOOTWEAR

It is important not only to select the correct type of shoes for exercise but also to replace them when they are worn. The three most common types of exercise shoe are cross trainers (multipurpose shoes), running shoes, and aerobics shoes.

Cross trainers are ideal if you work out in the gym, cycle, jog occasionally, and play racquet sports like badminton, but they are not recommended for high-impact aerobics.

Running shoes should be lightweight and have a wide, cushioned, elevated heel and good shock absorbency in the midsole to limit jarring of the ankle, knee, and hip joints. They should not be used for racquet sports because they do not provide sufficient support for the feet and ankles during sudden changes of direction.

Aerobics shoes should grip the floor firmly, have extra cushioning and shock absorbency in the toe to protect the ball of the foot during repeated impact, and provide ankle support. All workout shoes should be worn with thick socks to cushion the foot and prevent blisters. The best socks are made of cotton, to absorb perspiration, mixed with a little synthetic for shape retention. Some synthetic socks may look more absorbent than they actually are.

PREPARING YOUR BODY

A warm-up before exercise and a cool-down afterward will minimize the chance of injury and speed your body's recovery from the normal effects of a workout. Muscle fibers, tendons, and ligaments are more pliable at higher temperatures; by warming them up before exercise, you reduce the risk of incurring a strain or a sprain. A warm-up also helps increase your flexibility.

A number of physiological changes are believed to take place. For example, a warm-up causes the lungs to work more efficiently and, by raising blood and muscle temperature, makes the delivery of oxygen to the muscles more effective and increases the speed and efficiency of muscle contraction. A warm-up can further aid performance by preparing a person mentally for exercise.

After exercise it is very important to follow a cooling-down routine of simple movements that will slowly return the body to its pre-exercise state and get your heart and breathing rates back to normal gradually. Blood flow to the muscles increases during exercise; if you stop suddenly, the muscles will continue to receive a rapid blood supply that they no longer need. This can cause blood to pool in the legs, resulting in dizziness or fainting.

A GYM CHECKLIST

Make a checklist of what to take with you to the gym. Include:

▶ *Such clothing as shorts or a leotard, a T-shirt or sweatshirt, training shoes, sports socks.*

▶ *Water bottle.*

▶ *One towel for wiping perspiration off yourself and the equipment when you have finished and another towel for the shower.*

▶ *Flip-flops to wear in the shower.*

▶ *A comb, deodorant, and other toiletries.*

THE SPORTS SHOE

A sports shoe should be comfortable, well constructed, flexible, and most important, suitable for the activity and the surface on which it is to be used.

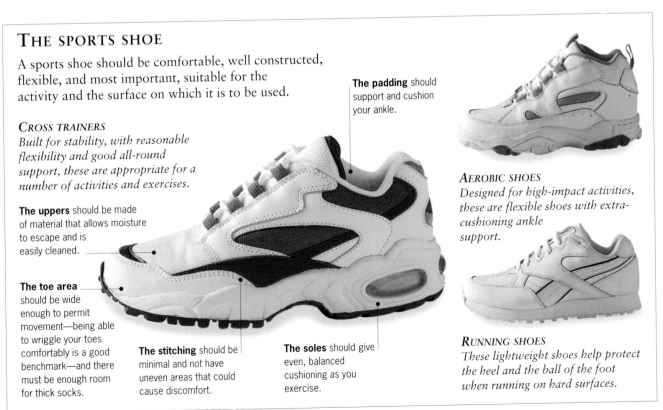

The padding should support and cushion your ankle.

CROSS TRAINERS
Built for stability, with reasonable flexibility and good all-round support, these are appropriate for a number of activities and exercises.

The uppers should be made of material that allows moisture to escape and is easily cleaned.

The toe area should be wide enough to permit movement—being able to wriggle your toes comfortably is a good benchmark—and there must be enough room for thick socks.

The stitching should be minimal and not have uneven areas that could cause discomfort.

The soles should give even, balanced cushioning as you exercise.

AEROBIC SHOES
Designed for high-impact activities, these are flexible shoes with extra-cushioning ankle support.

RUNNING SHOES
These lightweight shoes help protect the heel and the ball of the foot when running on hard surfaces.

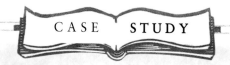

An Exercise Addict

Exercise addicts compulsively and obsessively work out, not necessarily to improve their fitness, health, or performance but to experience the buzz and adrenaline rush that accompany the effort. Exercise also provides relief from the negative feelings they experience when not working out and may become the center of their lives, to the exclusion of all else.

Linda is a 34-year-old graphic designer who initially took up exercise to lose a few pounds. She joined a local gym and enrolled in an aerobics class. When Linda first started, she exercised twice a week but somewhat to her surprise found herself enjoying the workouts so much that she began to do more and more. She now goes to the gym every evening after work, does one or more aerobic classes a day, and has started running on weekends. The more exercise Linda does, the more she wants to do. Exercising now takes up so much of her time that she has almost no other interests and is losing touch with her friends. She is often so exhausted that she finds it difficult to concentrate at work.

WHAT SHOULD LINDA DO?

Unless Linda slows down and reduces the amount of exercise she does, she is likely to injure herself or encounter other problems associated with overtraining. She needs to realize that while a moderate amount of exercise will keep her fit and healthy, her current exercise regimen is actually putting her health and emotional well-being at risk. She should limit the amount of time she puts aside for exercise each day and give herself easy exercise days, as well as complete rest days. Her exercise program should be flexible enough for her to miss a day and not feel guilty about it. She should then devote the additional free time to keeping in touch with friends and resuming old interests.

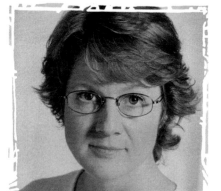

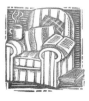

LIFESTYLE
The body needs time to recover from the demands that exercise places on it. Periods of rest and relaxation should be built into the daily lifestyle.

HEALTH
Too much exercise can result in increased vulnerability to illness and infection and susceptibility to injury, depression, and excessive weight loss.

EXERCISE
An intense exercise regimen that offers little flexibility can be physically and mentally damaging.

HOW THINGS TURNED OUT FOR LINDA

Linda has modified her attitude toward exercise. Although she still exercises regularly because she values and enjoys it, she now restricts the amount she does. She has built rest days into her program and reminds herself that she does not have to exercise every day. She now understands the importance of rest and feels much better for it. She has started French classes at night school and socializes regularly with her friends.

UNSAFE EXERCISES

When exercising, you must be fully confident that what you are doing and how you are doing it are safe. Surprisingly, some familiar exercises are potentially harmful to the body.

Some exercises are problematic not because they are inherently damaging but because they are often performed with poor technique. Generally speaking, they cause damage because they place too much stress on certain anatomical structures of the body, like the joints. It is important to realize that any exercise can lead to injury if it is performed incorrectly. For example, touching the toes with the legs straight or doing deep knee bends can be harmful.

Harmful or poorly executed exercises, if performed repeatedly on a regular basis, can cause immediate injury and/or long-term damage. The areas of your body that are particularly susceptible to harm are the neck, the knees, and the lower back.

PROBLEM ISSUES

Exercises that are likely to lead to injury are those in which the joints are subjected to extreme extension or arching, known as hyperextension, or extreme flexing or bending, called hyperflexion. Bouncing or flinging movements and stretches, continuous high-impact moves, and some isometric exercises can also be problematic and are inappropriate for many exercisers.

Ballistic work

Ballistic actions, such as swinging the arms vigorously from side to side, take muscles and other body structures rapidly to the end of their range of movement. Such movements can strain the muscles and place excessive demands on the joints, ligaments, and tendons.

These particular actions are often seen during warm-ups or aerobic dance or circuit sessions, but they are not advisable and can lead to such problems as muscle tears, as well as muscular stiffness and pain that could have been avoided. They can also overstretch the ligaments and result in

weakened joints and recurrent sprains. To avoid these problems, exercises should be performed at a controlled pace, and stretches should be held without bouncing.

Impact

Too much high-impact exercise places the joints under undue stress as they repeatedly absorb the body's weight on landing. This can be particularly problematic if the landings are poorly performed or are done on hard surfaces, such as concrete or wood. Whenever possible, high-impact activities should be interspersed with low-impact ones in which one foot always remains in contact with the ground.

Isometric work

Isometric exercises and weight training, in which there is tension in the muscles but little visible movement, have the potential to raise blood pressure; they should be done with caution or, in some cases, be avoided altogether. Isotonic exercises—in which the muscles can be seen to be working—are safer and more effective because they push the muscles through a wider range of movement (see page 130).

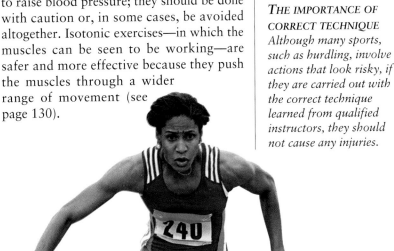

THE IMPORTANCE OF CORRECT TECHNIQUE Although many sports, such as hurdling, involve actions that look risky, if they are carried out with the correct technique learned from qualified instructors, they should not cause any injuries.

Exercising Safely

Any exercise can be harmful if done incorrectly. The correct ways to carry out some familiar and widely used exercises are shown here, together with some of the more common mistakes often made.

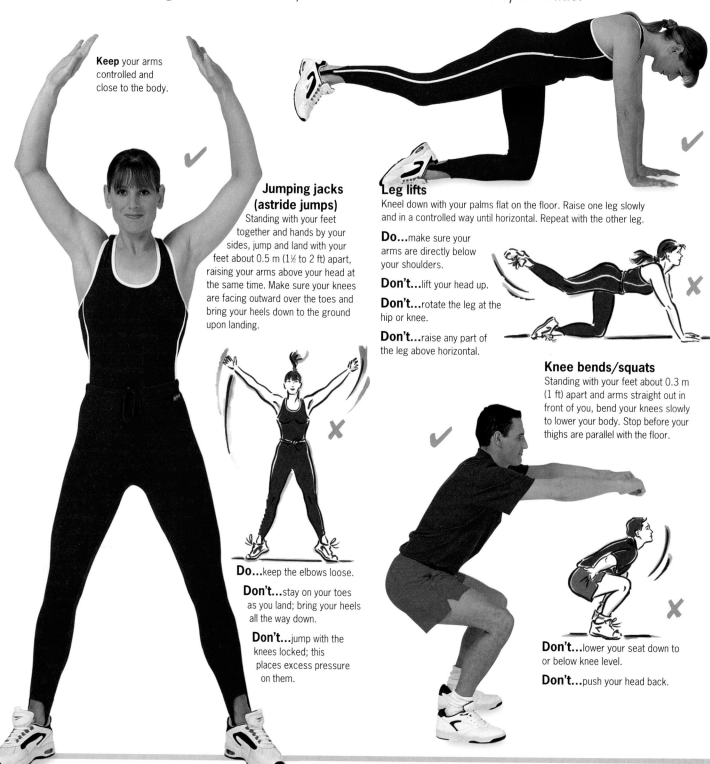

Keep your arms controlled and close to the body.

Jumping jacks (astride jumps)

Standing with your feet together and hands by your sides, jump and land with your feet about 0.5 m (1½ to 2 ft) apart, raising your arms above your head at the same time. Make sure your knees are facing outward over the toes and bring your heels down to the ground upon landing.

Do...keep the elbows loose.

Don't...stay on your toes as you land; bring your heels all the way down.

Don't...jump with the knees locked; this places excess pressure on them.

Leg lifts

Kneel down with your palms flat on the floor. Raise one leg slowly and in a controlled way until horizontal. Repeat with the other leg.

Do...make sure your arms are directly below your shoulders.

Don't...lift your head up.

Don't...rotate the leg at the hip or knee.

Don't...raise any part of the leg above horizontal.

Knee bends/squats

Standing with your feet about 0.3 m (1 ft) apart and arms straight out in front of you, bend your knees slowly to lower your body. Stop before your thighs are parallel with the floor.

Don't...lower your seat down to or below knee level.

Don't...push your head back.

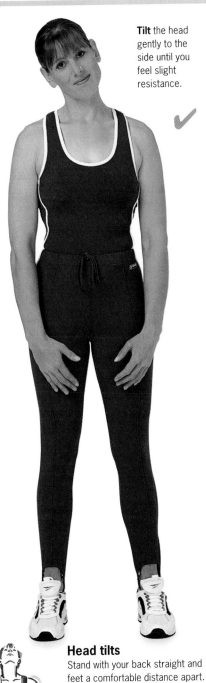

Tilt the head gently to the side until you feel slight resistance. ✔

Lunges

Starting with your feet shoulder width apart, step forward as far as you can comfortably manage and lower the rear leg to about 15 cm (6 in) from the floor. Draw your leading leg back and straighten up. Repeat, leading with the other leg.

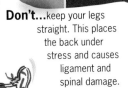

✔

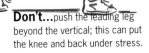 ✘

Don't...push the leading leg beyond the vertical; this can put the knee and back under stress.

Don't...lean forward. Keep your back straight and your upper body centered over your hips at all times.

Curl-ups

Lie on your back with knees bent, feet flat on the floor, and hands lightly touching your head. Breathe out as you slowly lift your shoulders off the floor. Keep your lower back on the floor and avoid using your hands to assist.

✔

Don't...keep your legs straight. This places the back under stress and causes ligament and spinal damage.

Don't...clasp your hands tightly behind your head. This causes the cervical spine to hyperflex, compressing the spinal discs and putting pressure on the nerves.

 ✘

Push-ups

Lie face down on the floor with hands directly under your shoulders, palms on the floor, and feet supported on your toes. Push your body off the floor until your arms are straight, supporting your lower body and legs on your toes, then lower your body again. Keep your back straight at all times.

✔

Head tilts

Stand with your back straight and feet a comfortable distance apart. Tilt your head to one side, then straighten it up. Repeat on the other side.

Don't...move the head in circles because this overextends and overflexes the neck and can damage the cervical spine and compress the nerve endings.

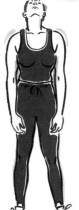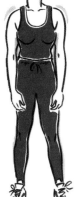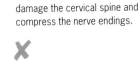 ✘

Don't...allow your hips and lower back to sag, which compresses the lower spine and can damage the spinal discs and back muscles.

Don't...tilt your head back or lock your elbows.

Don't...rest between push-ups.

 ✘

Sports injuries and remedies

With an understanding of the causes and effects of common sports injuries, you can treat some of them yourself and prevent them from occurring in the first place.

The most common physical disorders resulting from sports and exercise involve soft tissue damage. Such injuries affect the skin, muscles, tendons, or ligaments and include blisters, bruises, strains, sprains, cuts, and tears. The knees, shoulders, and elbows are the joints most frequently injured. And concussions from athletic activities are actually more common than once thought—some 330,000 a year occur throughout North America.

MUSCLE INJURIES

Soreness is the most common muscular complaint. There are two types: soreness felt during and immediately after exercise, and soreness and/or stiffness that usually does not appear until 24 to 48 hours later. The first type, associated with the accumulation of lactic acid following anaerobic exercise, usually passes quickly. The second is due to damaged muscle fibers and may last longer, depending on the extent of the damage.

In some injuries large numbers of muscle fibers may be torn, causing serious bleeding in the muscle. Painful swelling results, and movement is severely restricted. This kind of injury occurs through sudden overstretching or overreaching, often because insufficient time was spent warming up or stretching muscles beforehand. Lunging in racquet sports like tennis, for instance, or stopping abruptly and turning in sports such as soccer are common causes of torn muscles. A pulled muscle occurs for similar reasons but is a less serious injury, in which only a few muscle fibers are torn.

TENDON INJURIES

Overuse of a limb can lead to inflammation in the soft tissue surrounding the tendon. This is known as peritendinitis and causes the area to swell and become very tender. Tendinitis is an injury in which the tendon itself becomes inflamed, causing considerable pain. It most commonly affects the Achilles tendon, groin, or wrist.

A partial or complete rupture of a tendon can occur very suddenly under severe stress. The Achilles tendon and biceps are most often affected. Following a rupture you are unable to move the limb, and bleeding occurs in the gap between the split ends of

FOOT INJURIES

The foot is a complicated structure with ligaments, tendons, muscles and many small bones packed tightly together. Excess or repeated strain during exercise or sport can cause pain and injury and result in long-term weakening and instability, especially around the ankle joint.

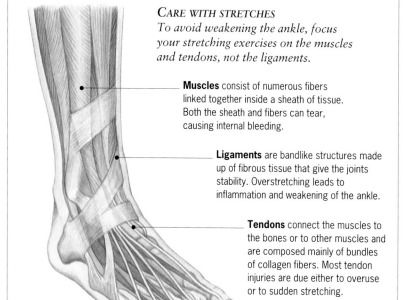

CARE WITH STRETCHES
To avoid weakening the ankle, focus your stretching exercises on the muscles and tendons, not the ligaments.

Muscles consist of numerous fibers linked together inside a sheath of tissue. Both the sheath and fibers can tear, causing internal bleeding.

Ligaments are bandlike structures made up of fibrous tissue that give the joints stability. Overstretching leads to inflammation and weakening of the ankle.

Tendons connect the muscles to the bones or to other muscles and are composed mainly of bundles of collagen fibers. Most tendon injuries are due either to overuse or to sudden stretching.

COMMON SPORTS INJURIES

This chart shows the 10 most common sports and exercise injuries revealed in a British survey; sprains and strains accounted for the largest percentage.

TYPE OF INJURY	PERCENTAGE
Sprains and strains	45.3
Unspecified pain and injury	21.9
Bruising	12.2
Cuts and scrapes	7.7
Illness	5.7
Tenderness, swelling, blisters	2.3
Dislocations	1.8
Fractures	1.8
Burns	1.1
Concussion	0.3

the tendon, which fills with blood and clots. A ruptured tendon is treated by resting and immobilizing the limb in a plaster cast.

LIGAMENT INJURIES

The ligaments commonly injured are in the knee and ankle joints. Such injuries most often occur when the joint is twisted through an abnormal range of movement or when excessive sideways pressure is exerted on it. This may result in a sprain, in which a few fibers are torn, or a complete tear, and usually causes severe pain and swelling.

OTHER INJURIES

Many other injuries can be avoided if consideration is given in advance to potential problems. For instance, if you are going to be doing a lot of running, consider the effect that the constant pounding on hard road surfaces will have on your limbs. Similarly, if you suffer from back problems, any training involving the back should be moderate or be avoided altogether.

Backache

Backache is common among exercisers and nonexercisers alike. However, when exercise involves excessive uncontrolled twisting, lifting, or contact, lower back pain may

result. As well as muscle tears and spasms or ligament tears, other common back complaints include prolapsed disc (slipped disc) and sciatica. A prolapsed disc occurs when an intervertebral disc ruptures and its gelatinous core seeps out, putting pressure on a nerve emerging from the spinal canal. The pain, which radiates down the leg as a result of a prolapsed disc, is known as sciatica. Although it can happen suddenly, it is usually the result of years of incorrect technique or overuse and not a direct result of the exercise you were doing at the time. Any exercise that puts undue stress on the back, especially if it is carried out incorrectly, can be the catalyst for injury.

Shin splints

This is the term commonly used to refer to pain down the front of the lower leg within the tibia. Shin splints can be caused by inflammation of the tendons, swelling of the muscles attached to the shin, or by a stress fracture. If caused by muscle swelling, shin splints may give rise to poor circulation and sometimes a feeling of numbness in the foot. Too much high-impact exercise, such as high-impact aerobics, or repetitive pounding on hard surfaces, as in road running, are common causes of shin splints.

REMEDIES FOR INJURIES

You can treat many exercise injuries yourself. You should, however, always consider whether they are serious enough to require professional help. If you feel a problem is something more than general aches and pains, pulled or strained muscles, or bruising, you should seek the advice of a doctor.

Basic first aid for injuries

For most types of acute injuries the treatment is the same. To treat bruises and tendon, muscle, and ligament injuries, use the four-stage RICE technique: Rest the injured limb; apply Ice to the injury; apply Compression; and Elevate the injured limb.

Treating an injury with RICE stops any bleeding and helps prevent swelling and inflammation, both of which can cause further tissue damage. It also ensures an early start to the healing process and promotes a quicker recovery while minimizing the risk of developing scar tissue and adhesions that might otherwise restrict movement of the injured limb in the future.

Minimizing post-exercise soreness
The soreness often experienced the day after strenuous exercise is sometimes referred to as delayed onset muscular soreness, or DOMS. While no measures can guarantee preventing DOMS completely, it can be minimized by warming up thoroughly prior to exercise and cooling down afterward. An adequate cooldown will help to dissipate lactic acid (a by-product of anaerobic exercise; see page 33) and maintain and develop flexibility in shortened muscles.

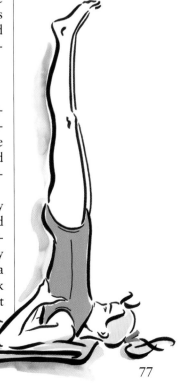

*NECK SUPPORT
The correct support during exercise can often minimize the risk of injury. For example, some yoga practitioners suggest placing a folded blanket or towel under the shoulders before doing the shoulder stand.*

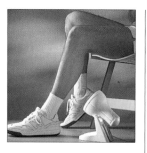

HOT STUFF
There are many types of heat lamps available for use at home today. They are useful for easing tense muscles, relieving general aches and pains, and speeding the repair of minor tissue damage. For more serious injuries, however, medical advice should be sought before using a heat lamp.

Rest is vital because continued use of an injured limb may increase bleeding, inflammation, or swelling and cause further damage.

Ice applied to an injury reduces pain by numbing the nerves and chilling the pain receptors. It also slows circulation of the blood, which stops bleeding and reduces inflammation and swelling. Ice should be applied for a maximum of 15 minutes at a time but can be reapplied every hour or so, once the limb warms up again. It may be necessary to continue ice treatment for one to two days following an injury.

Compression in the form of a bandage is applied to the injury to stop bleeding and help prevent swelling. A hard pad can be set over the injured area and a bandage then wrapped around it so that the pressure is concentrated on the damaged area.

Elevation of the injured limb should be done whenever possible to prevent pressure from gravity causing the limb to swell and increasing bleeding and inflammation.

Heat treatment

After the RICE technique has been applied, administering heat treatment by means of an infrared heat lamp, a heat pack, or a soaking bath can help to speed the repair of soft tissue damage, as well as relieve general aches and pains. Heat treatment can usually be applied two to three days after an injury, but it should not be used in the initial phase because it increases blood circulation, which can lead to more swelling and internal bleeding than would otherwise occur.

Heat increases blood flow to the affected area, which helps to wash away waste products and substances released by the damaged tissue. As waste products are removed, the tense muscles begin to relax, and pain is reduced. Heat also increases metabolism, which stimulates the repair processes in the body. Heat should not be applied for more than half an hour at a time, however, because tissue repair begins to suffer if a high temperature is maintained for too long.

NATURAL FIRST AID FOR SPORTS INJURIES

A well-stocked first-aid kit that combines natural remedies with conventional items can ease pain and speed recovery time. In addition to bandages, sterile strips, and cotton balls, petroleum jelly is useful and can be applied to prevent friction burns caused by clothing rubbing against the skin. You might include ibuprofen or aspirin to ease inflamed joints and acetaminophen for general pain relief.

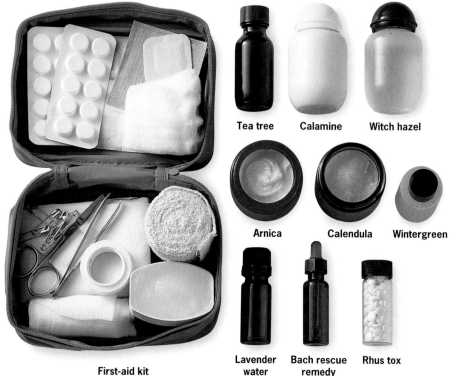

Tea tree   **Calamine**   **Witch hazel**

Arnica   **Calendula**   **Wintergreen**

Lavender water   **Bach rescue remedy**   **Rhus tox**

First-aid kit

Tea tree oil
is an antiseptic for minor cuts and grazes.

Calamine lotion
soothes bruises, abrasions, and friction burns.

Witch hazel
relieves blisters and friction burns.

Arnica cream
eases the pain of bruises and sprains.

Calendula cream
relieves inflammation and minor injuries.

Wintergreen oil
warms muscles and relieves muscle aches; it is also used to relieve blisters and friction burns.

Lavender water
soothes minor burns, sunburn, and headache.

Bach rescue remedy
can alleviate shock following an injury.

Rhus tox
is a homeopathic remedy used for cramps, sprains, and strains.

Treating a
Pulled Muscle

Strained muscles are one of the most common and easily sustained injuries, so it is worthwhile knowing how to deal with them. Although they are easy to treat, if you are at all unsure about the seriousness of the injury, you should see a doctor.

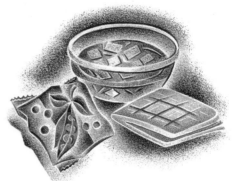

ALTERNATIVE ICE PACKS
To improvise an ice pack, use a packet of frozen peas wrapped in a dish towel or a compress soaked in a bowl of ice water.

The leg muscles are susceptible to pulls and strains, especially during exercise. A pulled muscle is felt as a sharp pain, and there is bleeding and discoloration visible under the skin. With appropriate treatment, the muscle will usually recover relatively quickly and heal within a couple of weeks. It is important to start light stretches as soon as possible to prevent scar tissue from forming, which may restrict movement in the muscle.

RICE – REST, ICE, COMPRESSION, ELEVATION

The immediate treatment for a pulled muscle is the application of RICE for at least 24 hours and preferably for longer, around two to three days.

After applying RICE to the injured leg, gentle movement and simple stretches can be started but keep within the limits of pain. Attempting to stretch or work the damaged muscle any sooner is likely to cause further pain and increase bleeding within the tissue, which will retard the healing process. It is usually possible to start gentle stretching exercises (see pages 126–7) when bruising appears on the surface of the skin. Over the next seven to ten days, gradually increase the amount of exercise you do. By this time a minor muscle tear should have repaired itself. If the muscle is still painful after a week or so, however, seek medical attention.

After recovery, continue to do stretches regularly in order to keep the muscle supple and prevent further injuries.

1 *Rest the leg and place as little weight on it as possible. You may want to use crutches to help the limb recover more quickly.*

2 *Apply an ice pack to the area and leave it in place for 5 to 15 minutes. Repeat the treatment every hour if necessary. To avoid ice burns, protect the skin by applying a layer of petroleum jelly and/or wrap a soft cloth around the ice pack.*

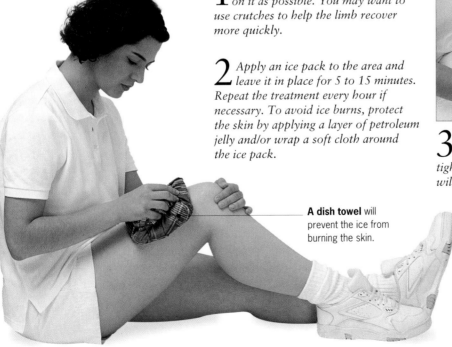

A dish towel will prevent the ice from burning the skin.

3 *Bind the damaged leg firmly with a bandage to compress it, but not so tightly that it stops your circulation. This will reduce the swelling.*

4 *The leg should be elevated to a level higher than your heart as often as possible, resting the limb on anything that is comfortable. This will reduce the pressure within the damaged blood vessels and thus reduce bleeding and inflammation.*

Medical help for concussion

A blow to the head that causes unconsciousness is known as concussion and is potentially very serious. A concussed person may feel sick and/or dizzy or have a headache. Never allow a person with a possible concussion to continue playing until seen by a doctor. If the person has been unconscious for more than 3 minutes or if there is blood or clear fluid seeping from the ears or nose, call an ambulance. Otherwise, get the person to rest, check him or her regularly, and seek medical help if the condition worsens.

Treatment can be repeated a little while after the temperature of the tissues has returned to normal.

Stretching

Sometimes excess tension in the muscles can contribute to or even cause an injury, as well as slow down the recovery process. Static stretching can reduce the tension in the muscle (see pages 126–127) and aid recovery. As with heat treatment, stretching should not be done immediately after an injury occurs because it can lead to more swelling and internal bleeding. After a few days of rest, however, stretching will help to speed up the healing process.

Perform stretches only when the muscles are warm. Ease into them slowly and then hold still. You should feel mild tension in the muscle while stretching, but there should not be any pain.

Self-massage

Self-massage can be useful in treating injuries and in reducing muscle tension. However, this technique is not recommended during the first two or three days after an injury. When you practice self-massage, you become aware of muscle tension in the area dissipating, and you can use this treatment whenever you feel tension building up. The benefits of self-massage are the same as for massage that is performed by others, although not all techniques can be performed the same way.

You can make an herbal massage cream with infused oils from such herbs and spices as cayenne pepper or mustard or try the soothing massage oil described below. These oils warm the muscles and ease away tension, aches, and pains.

Liniments and ointments

Liniments and ointments for the relief of sports injuries usually contain substances that act as an irritant to the skin and cause dilation of blood vessels near the surface. This action in turn causes blood to be diverted to the skin from the deeper tissues, thus creating a sensation of warmth and helping to relieve pain.

Ingredients most often found in liniments and ointments include salicylic acid, nicotinic acid, Spanish pepper (capsaicin) and etheric oils, such as turpentine or menthol. Some of these ingredients are allergenic, which means they may cause allergic reactions in some people. If you have sensitive or broken skin, you should look for products labeled hypoallergenic.

MAKING YOUR OWN MASSAGE OIL FOR ACHING MUSCLES

Making a massage oil for the relief of muscle aches is simple, requiring few ingredients and little time or effort. By combining the essential oils of herbs such as comfrey or chamomile (available from herbal suppliers and some drug stores), which stimulate cell repair; rosemary or eucalyptus to aid circulation; and the infused oil of St. John's wort to reduce any minor swelling, you can create a relaxing rub to soothe your muscular aches and pains.

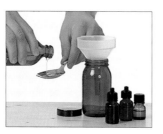

2 Before each massage, shake the jar well. Warm the oil by rubbing a little between your hands before applying it to the muscle. Reapply when the oil gets absorbed into the skin.

1 Slowly combine 250 ml (9 fl oz) of St. John's wort infused oil with the essential oils of chamomile (5 ml, or 100 drops), eucalyptus (2 ml, or 40 drops), and comfrey (1 ml, or 20 drops) in a glass jar.

Massage the oil into the muscles using gentle, smooth, sweeping movements to begin with, making the strokes firmer as the muscles warm up.

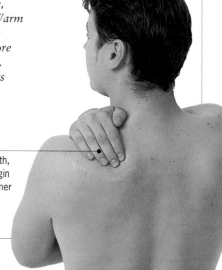

TREATING INJURIES PROFESSIONALLY

You may sustain an injury during exercise that is too severe for self-treatment. If this should happen, it helps to know what type of professional help you require.

With an injury or exercise-induced illness, it is important to know when to consult your doctor or seek emergency aid and when you can safely treat yourself. If you suspect a fracture, avoid movement to prevent further damage. When a limb is broken, movement of it will be difficult and it may be badly swollen or hanging at an unusual angle. If in doubt, treat the injury as a fracture.

Some kinds of pain that arise during or immediately after exercise are warning signals that you need attention by a doctor. These signals include pain that gets steadily worse and that is accompanied by other symptoms, such as vomiting, dizziness, pins and needles, tingling, numbness, or any other unusual persistent symptoms. Once an acute injury has been treated, the doctor may refer you to other specialists for further treatment and rehabilitation.

Physiotherapy
Physiotherapy involves the use of injury-specific progressive exercise combined with various treatments to facilitate rapid tissue repair and the restoration of full mobility. The particular form of treatment will depend on the type and severity of the injury and how long ago is was sustained. Common treatments include cold, heat, ultrasound (deep heat therapy using high-frequency sound waves), electrical stimulation, massage, manipulations, and exercise.

Osteopathy and chiropractic
Osteopathy and chiropractic involve the use of manipulative techniques to release mechanical blocks in the musculoskeletal system (freeing a locked joint, for example); break down adhesions that are preventing a full range of movement; and repositioning damaged spinal disc material. The manipulations are usually performed at the sites of joint injuries. The joint is taken to the end of its current range of motion, and then the practitioner applies a quick thrust to free the blockage. These actions require a high degree of skill and should be performed only by qualified practitioners.

Massage
Massage can be used in both the prevention and treatment of injury. It can help reduce muscle soreness and pain, break down scar tissue to restore muscle integrity and full range of movement, and promote overall relaxation. Gentle massage can usually be applied to muscle strains two to three days

continued on page 84

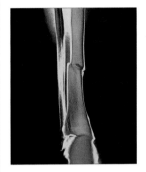

HAVE IT EXAMINED
If there is a possibility that an injury might involve a fracture, seek professional help. If left to set by themselves, even minor fractures can mend out of alignment.

UNDERSTANDING NEEDS
A physiotherapist will encourage a patient with a damaged joint to exercise it as soon as possible after the injury to ensure that the healing process does not lead to restricted movement. The injury may have to be monitored for weeks, months, or even years, depending on its severity, to make sure there are no lasting flexibility problems.

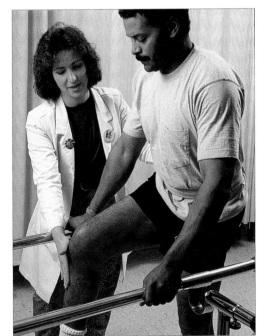

Sports Physiotherapist

No matter how fit or experienced you are in your chosen discipline, all exercises and sports carry the risk of injury. If an injury is serious and cannot be treated by yourself or your doctor, you may need the services of a sports physiotherapist.

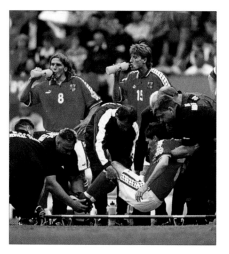

SPEEDY ASSISTANCE
Muscular injuries, which are common in competitive team play, require fast and effective action. A sports physiotherapist who is on hand throughout a game can act immediately in case of injury.

Origins

The roots of physiotherapy can be traced back to the medicinal massage techniques practiced in ancient times. But it was not until 1894, when the Society of Trained Masseuses was formed in Britain, that the discipline first gained public recognition.

The society was founded by four young nurses and midwives, largely to distinguish medicinal massage from the illicit massage parlors prevalent at the time. During its early years men were ineligible to join the society or to receive therapeutic massage. However, an influx of casualties from the First World War led to a change, and by 1920, when the society was granted a royal charter, men were being accepted as both patients and members. The organization is now known

Sports physiotherapy emerged from the more general practice of physiotherapy. Sports therapists specialize in the treatment of professional and amateur athletes, although they also treat members of the general public who have sustained a sports-related injury.

What do sports physiotherapists do?

Primarily they treat sports injuries, but they also supply training and exercise advice for patients until they

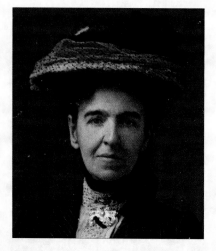

ROSALIND PAGET
Miss (later Dame) Rosalind Paget, a midwife, was the first chairperson of the Society of Trained Masseuses.

as The Chartered Society of Physiotherapy and has proved the therapeutic worth of physiotherapy to generations of sick and injured people.

are able to participate fully in their sport again. Sports physiotherapists also provide first aid when an injury occurs and are involved in every stage of the healing process until recovery. They have special knowledge of injury treatment and prevention and an awareness of exercise physiology, sports psychology, and sports medicine. They also act as liaison between the patient and medical and surgical specialists, as well as other paramedic practitioners.

Who else do sports physiotherapists consult?

This depends on the nature of the patient's injury and activities. A sports physiotherapist often acts as liaison with orthopedic surgeons, who specialize in treating disorders of the bones and joints; podiatrists, who are concerned with disorders of the feet and lower limbs, particularly those that affect normal walking; dietitians; sports psychologists; exercise physiologists; paramedics; masseurs; coaches; trainers; physical education teachers; managers; promoters; parents of young athletes; sometimes the media; and other health practitioners. A cardiac specialist, for instance, might be called in to treat an athlete who has developed a heart disorder, perhaps as a result of overtraining.

Where do they practice?

Sports physiotherapists work in hospitals, group medical practices, rehabilitation centers, physiotherapy clinics, and health centers. They also work for health clubs and fitness centers. Some are hired by athletic teams to look after the total needs of its members, including preseason conditioning at training camp and the care and rehabilitation of injuries.

What sort of injuries do they treat?

Sports physiotherapists treat the whole range of musculoskeletal problems, from bruises, strains, and sprains to joint, spinal, and head injuries. They also help deal with mobility problems from inflammation and repetitive strain injury. A significant proportion of their work, however, is injury prevention, which involves advising athletes on correct stretching and warm-up procedures and ways to avoid techniques that can be damaging or risky.

What methods and equipment do they use?

Many approaches may be used as part of general physiotherapy practice, including massage and manipulation, electrotherapy, hydrotherapy, ultrasound, lasers, heat and cold therapies, traction, acupuncture, relaxation techniques, and exercise therapy. Your therapist should be aware of your physical fitness needs and should be able to combine your fitness training schedules with remedial exercise treatment for your injury.

How long has sports physiotherapy been around?

The practice has been around since the 1950s, but formal accreditation of physiotherapists to deal specifically with sports injuries began in the 1970s, when televised international events like the Olympic Games produced an unprecedented rise in public interest in athletics. Important breakthroughs in sports medicine and technology also encouraged this momentum. By the arrival of the fitness boom in the mid-1980s, sports physiotherapy was well established.

How do I choose a practitioner?

A physiotherapist who is a member of the American Physical Therapy Association (APTA), which is based in Alexandria, Virginia, will have met the educational requirements listed below. The association does not make referrals, however.

In Canada you can contact your provincial branch of the Canadian Physiotherapy Association or Sports Physiotherapy Canada in Gloucester, Ontario, for a recommendation.

What training is required?

Sports physiotherapy is one of several subspecialties of the practice. Practitioners must have a university degree in physiotherapy, have completed a clinical internship, done at least 800 hours of postgraduate work involving a variety of sports injuries and problems, and passed a special examination.

What can I expect from my first visit?

Your physiotherapist will examine the injury, take note of how and when it occurred, and provide some initial remedial treatment. He or she may also prescribe some exercises for you to perform on your own, which will aid tissue repair, restore joint mobility, and help ensure that the muscles do not weaken through prolonged inactivity.

WHAT YOU CAN DO AT HOME

A physiotherapist's skills can do much to speed the healing process, but measures you take on your own will play a vital part in ensuring a full recovery. For example, you should rest an injured limb at first but should begin a planned program of exercises to regain flexibility in the joints and strengthen the muscles as soon as a physiotherapist gives you the go ahead. In addition, you should maintain a well-balanced diet. Protein-rich foods are important for tissue repair; extra calcium may be needed to promote a strong repair of a broken bone; and such foods as oily fish and garlic have been found to be beneficial in reducing inflammation.

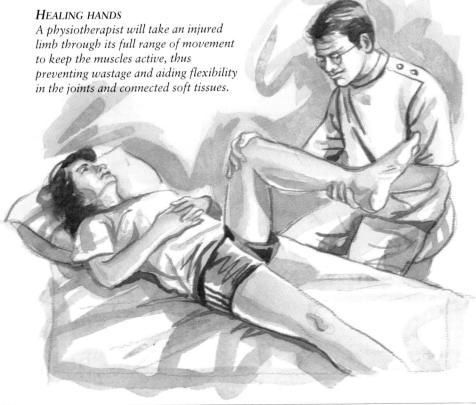

HEALING HANDS
A physiotherapist will take an injured limb through its full range of movement to keep the muscles active, thus preventing wastage and aiding flexibility in the joints and connected soft tissues.

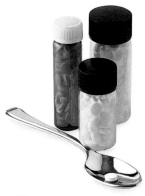

HOMEOPATHIC REMEDIES
Homeopaths recommend several remedies for exercise-related injuries. These include Rhus tox *for muscular strains and cramps,* Ruta grav *for aching bones and muscles, and* Arnica *for bruising and shock.*

after the injury, and with mild or moderate strains, deep massage can usually begin after seven days. Massage restores the circulation, helping to reduce muscle tightness and improve tissue elasticity, flexibility, tone, and overall muscle balance.

Aromatherapy

The use of essential oils as preventive and curative treatments has become a popular form of therapy. The oils, each of which has special properties and benefits, are extracted from flowers, leaves, fruit, bark, roots, and/or wood, and can be used for a variety of conditions. Aromatherapy oils are best applied through massage or compresses or added to bathwater. When using aromatherapy oils for massage, always mix them with a base, such as almond oil, first.

Acupuncture/acupressure

Age-old healing techniques from the Orient, acupuncture and acupressure involve locating channels and pressure points in the body that are believed to contain and control the flows of energy that course through the

Pathway to health

Because there is such a wide choice of complementary therapies to choose from, you should be able to find one that is appropriate to your injury or symptoms and convenient for you. This may mean combining one or two different treatments. Backache, for example, can be temporarily relieved by hydrotherapy or massage, but you might also want to see an osteopath to get to the root of the problem. Always follow all instructions carefully when preparing any treatment for yourself or others and, if in any doubt, seek help from a specialist.

body. Stimulating the points by inserting needles (acupuncture) or by applying pressure (acupressure) influences the energy flow. Both can be used to relieve pain, fatigue, and muscle tension and encourage healing of bruising, fractures, and sprains.

Hydrotherapy

Hydrotherapy involves the use of water for treatment and rehabilitation. Whirlpool and other baths, water jets, hot and cold showers, and massage are among the tools of hydrotherapy that are used to tackle a range of common injuries. Hydrotherapy is particularly beneficial when there is limited movement, temporary muscle weakness, impaired coordination, or a diminished sense of balance following an injury. The buoyancy of water relieves the stresses of weight bearing on joints, while warm water relieves muscle pain or spasm and helps to reduce bruising and swelling by increasing circulation. Swelling is also reduced by the pressure of water on the affected area.

Homeopathy

Homeopaths do not advocate supplanting any methods of orthodox or manipulative therapy, but do recommend homeopathic remedies in place of orthodox drugs because the homeopathic ones produce no undesirable side effects. Homeopathy is believed to provide relief from shock and pain and to be effective in helping the body heal sprains, fractures, and other injuries. Various general remedies are available from pharmacies and health food stores.

SHIATSU

Shiatsu is a form of soft tissue manipulation that can be used to induce muscular and general relaxation, speed recovery after an injury, and treat specific injuries and illnesses. Its origins lie in ancient Eastern therapeutic techniques, but it was not developed into a comprehensive therapy until early in the 20th century. As with acupressure, the fingers and thumbs are used to manipulate acupuncture points. However, a shiatsu therapist may also use the knee, shin, and foot to apply stronger pressure.

HEALING TOUCH
Shiatsu can help to enhance relaxation and concentration before an exercise session and aid muscle recovery and tissue repair afterward.

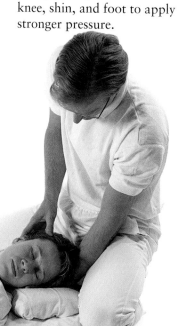

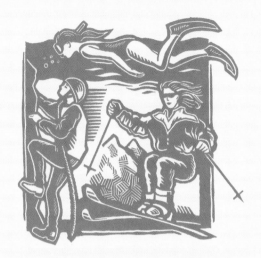

SPORTS FOR FUN AND FITNESS

*There is such a vast range of sports
and other active pursuits to choose from,
you should easily find one or more to suit you.
Before making a choice, however, think about
your fitness goals, the demands of your
lifestyle, and whether you have to take
any health problems into account.*

SPORT CHOICES FOR ALL AGES

Many factors may play a part in determining your choice of a physical activity. You have to consider your health, age, skills, lifestyle, and fitness goals—and what you enjoy doing.

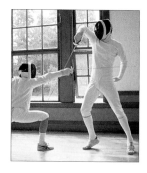

AGELESS EXERCISE
Such sports as fencing are accessible to people of all ages. They require more suppleness and mobility than strength and stamina.

Age does not have to dictate the choice of sports activities for you or your family, but every age group has particular needs that should be considered when making a decision. If you have a family, think about ways in which you can involve all the members for at least some of your active pursuits. For example, if you have young children, playing games with them can be good exercise for all of you. In the same way, think about involving your own parents in an exercise plan or choosing some activities for both grandchildren and grandparents. Family exercise can help strengthen relationships, as well as improve everybody's fitness and general health.

Children

For younger children the focus should be on fun. Try not to overwhelm small children with the complexities of organized sports too soon; playing tag and simple games with a ball and splashing in a swimming pool are great exercises for them. Cycling and hiking are fine for youngsters over the age of seven. As children grow older, team games help them to develop social skills and at the same time learn to interact with others and to accept and respect the need for rules.

You can encourage children to participate in physical activities instead of watching television or playing computer games by enrolling them in a community center or

---

A HEALTHY LIFESTYLE

Whatever sport you choose, the most important point to remember is that it should be part of a healthy lifestyle.

Make sure that your body has adequate rest and nutrition to cope with the increased demands being placed on it.

ADEQUATE SLEEP
Get as much rest as your body needs and try to maintain regular sleep and waking times.

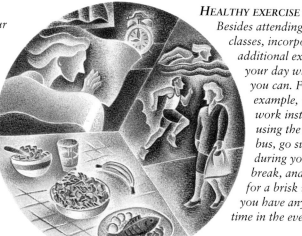

HEALTHY EXERCISE
Besides attending fitness classes, incorporate additional exercise into your day whenever you can. For example, walk to work instead of using the car or bus, go swimming during your lunch break, and jog or go for a brisk walk if you have any free time in the evening.

BALANCED DIET
Have at least three meals a day and never skip a meal. Make sure your diet includes plenty of fresh fruits and vegetables and starchy carbohydrates.

DEVELOPMENT OF SPORTING SKILLS

Children enjoy games from an early age, but their approach changes over time as their coordination and skills improve. It is important to bear this in mind when encouraging children to play physical games so they will stay motivated.

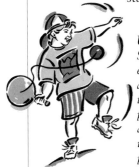

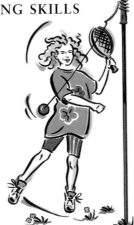

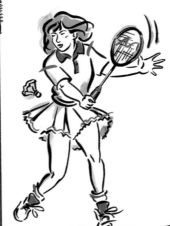

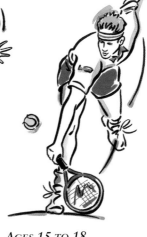

UNDER 8
Small children enjoy simple bat and ball games that they can play on their own and improve on with regular practice.

AGES 8 TO 11
Games that can be played with friends help keep older children interested.

AGES 12 TO 14
Young teenagers are best motivated by games that require high skill levels.

AGES 15 TO 18
Older teenagers often need a strong element of competition in their sport.

club that offers sports for them to explore. Remember, however, that young children subjected to intensive training may suffer injuries and disappointments. Being pushed too hard can actually lower their self-esteem and discourage them from taking part in sports instead of encouraging them in an active, healthy lifestyle. Try to make sure that exercise is fun and a little bit challenging and don't place undue pressure on children to exceed their capabilities.

Teenagers

During puberty boys tend to become more physically adept and capable at sports, while girls sometimes find that the changes in their bodies add challenges that discourage them from participating. Girls who have taken up sports like gymnastics, for which a small physique to facilitate quick, dainty movements is an advantage, may find that particular sport no longer possible after puberty. These teenagers need to be encouraged to find other activities in which they can continue to use and enjoy the skills they have learned. For example, dance can be a good choice for a former gymnast because it utilizes many of the coordination skills already learned in gymnastics.

Some teenagers give up a particular sport because of pressure to excel from parents, teachers, or coaches. In such cases they should be encouraged to try different sports, especially noncompetitive ones, or to participate at a level that challenges without overwhelming them. Summer camps provide multiple activities for teenagers and may help them to discover a new type of activity that they can enjoy. Encouraging teenagers to walk or cycle rather than driving them everywhere can also increase their exercise levels considerably, although considerations of safety obviously come first.

Young adults

Many people find that the opportunity and desire to participate in sports and regular exercise dissipates after leaving school, especially when facilities become less readily accessible. Many jobs force people into a more sedentary lifestyle than they knew at school, and starting a family can leave little time for exercise and sporting pursuits.

Although you may want to return to a sport you once enjoyed in your teens, you may find that you are no longer fit enough. Follow the adage: "Get fit to play sports—don't play sports to get fit." For those who have been inactive for some years, a gradual reintroduction to exercise, followed by a steady buildup, is important.

Keep lifestyle in mind as well; if stress, anxiety, or depression is a factor in your life, it may be helpful to think about activities that could alleviate it. For example, if you feel under constant pressure at work, a relaxing form of exercise, such as yoga, may meet your needs. Parents may have to choose an activity that they can do while the children are in play groups or at school.

A Disappointed Dancer

Rapid physical change during puberty can mean that activities once suitable for a girl are no longer appropriate for a full-figured teenager. Many girls attend classical ballet classes, only to find that they no longer meet ballet's standards once they gain their adult height and build. However, with family encouragement and support, they needn't cease to be active altogether.

Sylvie is a 15-year-old student living at home with her parents and younger sister, Jane. Until age 13 Sylvie was a keen student of ballet, but last year it became obvious that she was going to be too tall and well built to become a classical ballet dancer. Sylvie loves dancing and was very upset to give up her girlhood ambition. To make matters worse, her younger sister is still taking ballet lessons, and she teases Sylvie about her new figure and the fact that she no longer dances. Thinking that if she's going to be big she may as well eat what she likes and not worry about her figure, Sylvie takes comfort in sweets. This, combined with lack of exercise, is contributing to a weight problem.

WHAT SHOULD SYLVIE DO?

Sylvie has to find a form of exercise that can be adapted to her former interests and skills. There are plenty of other activities that involve music and movement and aren't so restrictive in terms of body shape. She needs support from her family, not teasing. Her parents should help her find alternative outlets for dancing skills and encourage her to change her diet, reducing her consumption of sweets and reorienting her toward healthier options. Sylvie's mother should also help her daughter become comfortable with the rapid physical changes that have taken place; shopping together for clothes that flatter Sylvie's new shape could be a confidence booster.

Action Plan

DIET
Make sure that your diet is well balanced, with lots of fruits and vegetables rather than fatty or high-sugar snack foods.

EMOTIONAL HEALTH
Talk through any worries you have about your lifestyle or appearance. You may find a great deal of support and understanding from family and friends.

EXERCISE
Find alternatives to pastimes you have outgrown. Many skills learned in one physical activity can be applied to others.

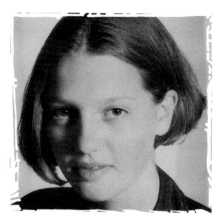

DIET
High-calorie comfort foods offer only short-term relief and can exacerbate a problem with weight or body shape.

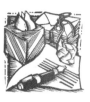

EMOTIONAL HEALTH
Feelings of embarrassment and inadequacy due to adolescent changes in the body can cause sadness and fear in young people.

EXERCISE
Suddenly giving up exercise can have an immediate and detrimental effect on fitness and body shape.

HOW THINGS TURNED OUT FOR SYLVIE

Sylvie's mother encouraged her to take up flamenco dancing as an alternative to ballet. Initially skeptical, Sylvie soon found that the dramatic style of flamenco reawakened her interest in performing. She began paying closer attention to her diet and substituting sweets with low-fat energy foods, such as bananas. Sylvie found that her return to dancing improved her self-confidence, and she's now content with her new figure.

Middle age

Middle age is a period during which many people decide to take up exercise for the first time in a long while. Often an increase in weight or a medical checkup prompts this decision. Regular exercise helps combat the stresses of work and home life, prevent weight gain, and slow physical decline. For example, the risk of osteoporosis can be lessened by undertaking weight-bearing exercises, such as walking and aerobics, which help maintain bone mass.

It is generally better to choose an activity that fits in with your lifestyle rather than rearrange your lifestyle to fit around your choice of exercise. If you are a busy executive, for instance, you may be able to fit in exercise only before work, and the program will have to be as time efficient as possible.

Most experts recommend starting with a gentle form of exercise, like walking, to build up your aerobic fitness. Monitor improvements in your heart rate and, as your basic level of fitness improves, think next about any special fitness requirements of your favorite sport. For example, some degree of suppleness is required for racquet sports, so flexibility training will help to make a return to these sports much easier. You could also look for clubs that run sections specifically for training and competition of older players.

Old age

Some physical decline in old age is inevitable. However, severe disability can be as much a result of inactivity as of aging itself. Research shows that strength can be not only maintained but actually improved in old age and that this improvement is associated with an increase in bone density, which also helps to stave off osteoporosis.

Stamina and flexibility can be improved as well, allowing older people more freedom of movement and a greater vitality and ability to enjoy life. Further studies have shown that the slowing in reaction times that often occurs in sedentary older people is not so marked in those who take steps to remain physically active.

Walking, swimming, moderate weight training, exercise to music, and dancing are all appropriate forms of exercise for the older adult. For those who have remained actively involved in a sport, continued participation in that sport is possible, provided

---

EXERCISE ON VACATION

Try not to neglect exercise while on vacation, or it may be difficult to get back into a fitness routine when you return. At the beach, in addition to sunbathing, play volleyball or swim for 10 minutes every hour. Walk on the deepest parts of the sand, which will make your legs work harder. Jog on the beach in the early morning, before the sun gets too hot, or late in the afternoon. Contact a local hiking group, cycle touring club, or mountain bike club to see if there are any events you can participate in during your stay, or take advantage of snorkeling, water skiing, or windsurfing facilities.

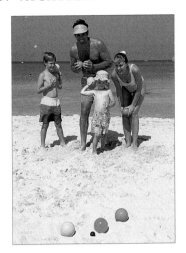

FAMILY FUN
Encourage your children to play ball games, Frisbee, or beach volleyball and join them in play.

---

there are no precluding health problems. For the frail elderly, improvements in strength, stamina, and flexibility will enhance their quality of life, but their exercise should always be supervised by instructors with special training.

For many old people a lack of independence is linked to a loss of ability to cope with everyday tasks, such as washing their own hair, walking upstairs, or getting in and out of a bathtub unaided. Much of this loss of ability is related to a reduction in strength and power, which in itself is associated with a decrease in muscle mass, bone density, and balance. Therefore, for older adults muscular strength work is a keystone to an active and independent retirement.

Remember, though, that if you have a particular health problem, it is important to discuss exercise options with a doctor or sports physiotherapist. This is because various forms of exercise tax different parts of the body, so you need to be sure you are choosing one that will be of most benefit without overstressing weak areas. For example, if you suffer from asthma, an activity like swimming in an indoor pool, which strengthens lung capacity in a warm environment that is less likely to trigger an attack, is of particular benefit. Swimming is also beneficial if you suffer from arthritis because water supports your weight, allowing movement without stressing the joints.

CHOOSING A SPORT

Understanding what level of fitness is needed for a particular sport, what equipment is necessary, and how the sport is likely to benefit your health will help you choose the right one.

ADVENTURE SPORTS
Adventure sports are outdoor leisure activities that combine a high degree of skill and physical effort with an element of risk. They appeal to people who enjoy the challenge of pushing themselves to the limit, both physically and mentally. Adventure sports have strict safety rules that should be adhered to at all times, and all require strict training under expert supervision to keep risks within acceptable limits.

You don't have to be the athletic type to participate in sports. There is such a wide range of physical activities available, you should be able to find one that meets your particular needs, whether you are looking for a low-key activity that includes socializing, some outdoor fun, a physical challenge, or something that allows your creativity full rein.

When choosing a sport, it is important to take into account such personal factors as temperament, commitment, and individual skills. For example, some people are happiest when playing as part of a team, while others prefer sports that require self-reliance and individual skill and flare.

Similarly, some sports may require a greater commitment in terms of financial outlay, practice sessions, or training than you are prepared to give. By choosing an activity you will enjoy and that fits into your lifestyle, you will find it easier to maintain your motivation and achieve your fitness goals. No matter which sport appeals to you, age need not be a barrier. Opportunities abound for people of all ages to take part in a great many sports.

MAKING YOUR CHOICE

To help you choose a sporting activity that best suits your abilities, interests, and personal aspirations, the following pages feature a number of sports and describe their requirements in terms of costs, skills, time, fitness, and equipment. Some of the activities featured, including walking, running, and swimming, will suit the solitary exerciser who wants to fit the activity into a busy life. Other sports are for those who prefer the camaraderie and competitiveness of team play or racquet sports. This chapter also focuses on particular skills you will

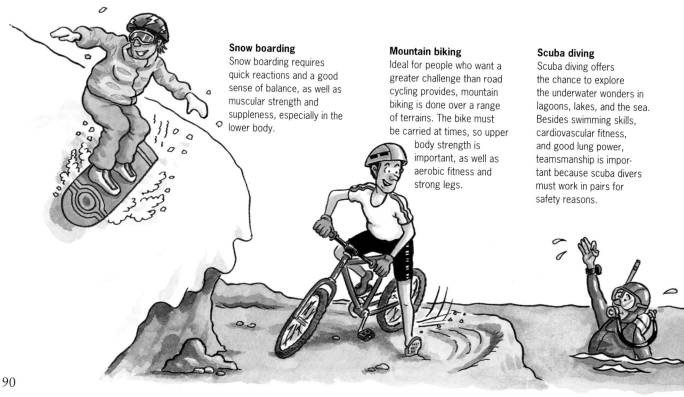

Snow boarding
Snow boarding requires quick reactions and a good sense of balance, as well as muscular strength and suppleness, especially in the lower body.

Mountain biking
Ideal for people who want a greater challenge than road cycling provides, mountain biking is done over a range of terrains. The bike must be carried at times, so upper body strength is important, as well as aerobic fitness and strong legs.

Scuba diving
Scuba diving offers the chance to explore the underwater wonders in lagoons, lakes, and the sea. Besides swimming skills, cardiovascular fitness, and good lung power, teamsmanship is important because scuba divers must work in pairs for safety reasons.

need in order to get the most from the sport and other exercises you can do specifically to improve the degree of fitness and muscular strength required.

If you are interested in any of the team sports, one way to get started is to see if they are featured in the sports pages or classified sections of your local newspaper; many teams advertise locally for new players. Or check out work-based sports and social clubs. You could also ask at your local library, church hall, or sports or community center. Don't be put off by the need for special equipment. Many organizations will lend or rent equipment to beginners or players who participate only occasionally.

FIT TO PLAY

In all sports, getting fit before you play ensures better performance, a lower risk of injury, and greater enjoyment. Fatigue, in particular, is the enemy of good performance. Once tired, you will lose strength, speed, skill, and concentration and become injury prone.

For sports that require multiple sprints—soccer and basketball, for example—basic aerobic fitness is important, and this can be acquired through regular walking, running, or jogging. Many sports require a combination of different types of fitness, such as flexibility, muscular strength, and endurance. These can be achieved by combining resistance or circuit training with aerobic activities. Different sports also place their own unique demands on the body. The physical demands of a fast and furious game of ice hockey, for instance, are vastly different from those of a tennis match or a day-long hike. It follows that each sport requires its own type of fitness training, coupled with the right mental outlook, for players to get the most benefits from the game.

Contact sports such as football and judo require overall muscular strength to withstand tackles and throws. Horseback riding calls for balance and muscular endurance to remain in the saddle and in control as the horse canters, gallops, or jumps. Swimming and gymnastics require flexibility combined with strength and stamina.

People participating in sports should prepare with a good stretch and warm-up routine, just as they would for any other type of exercise. At the end of a game, they should stretch thoroughly, paying particular attention to the hamstrings and hip flexors.

You can take up any sport you choose, as long as you are reasonably fit and have no medical conditions that may impair your performance or put your health at greater than normal risk. If you have diabetes, epilepsy, angina, asthma, or high blood pressure, have had recent surgery, or are pregnant, consult your doctor before deciding on any new activity.

POPULAR PURSUITS
Surveys have revealed that walking is by far the most popular way to keep fit in North America. Also high on the list are swimming, social dancing, gardening, and cycling.

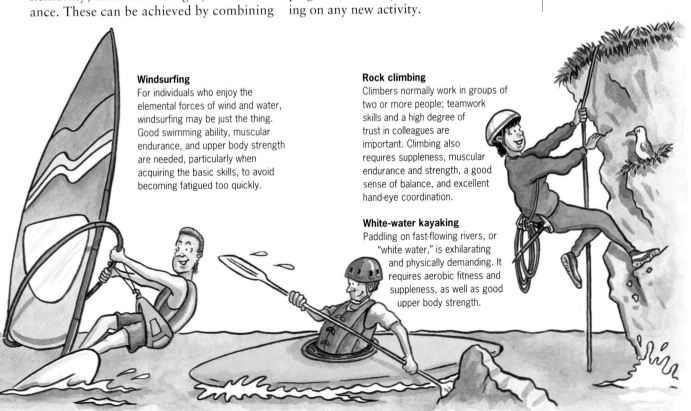

Windsurfing
For individuals who enjoy the elemental forces of wind and water, windsurfing may be just the thing. Good swimming ability, muscular endurance, and upper body strength are needed, particularly when acquiring the basic skills, to avoid becoming fatigued too quickly.

Rock climbing
Climbers normally work in groups of two or more people; teamwork skills and a high degree of trust in colleagues are important. Climbing also requires suppleness, muscular endurance and strength, a good sense of balance, and excellent hand-eye coordination.

White-water kayaking
Paddling on fast-flowing rivers, or "white water," is exhilarating and physically demanding. It requires aerobic fitness and suppleness, as well as good upper body strength.

Sports for Fitness

Walking, running, swimming, and cycling all provide a solid basis for fitness and are probably the best activities to choose if you have been inactive for some time. Their levels of intensity can be increased as your fitness improves.

WALKING

Walking is a low-impact, weight-bearing activity that places less stress on the joints than many other forms of exercise. There are more forms of walking than many people imagine, but all will improve aerobic fitness and tone the muscles of the lower body—and the upper body to some extent. If you have been inactive for a while, walking is an excellent way to regain fitness, but you should start slowly and build up gradually.

Walking faster, farther, uphill, or on rough terrain increases the intensity of a walk and is therefore

> Walking requires little equipment and can be tailored to suit the fitness levels and needs of anyone. It improves stamina and—if a gradient is included—also builds strength.

more demanding. When starting a walking program, assess the activity you do on a regular basis and begin your walking regimen just above this level. For example, if you normally walk for just 10 minutes to and from the bus stop every day, you will have to improve your general fitness level before attempting a full day's ramble or a hike up steep hills.

Getting started

Plan your route before you start. Whenever possible, avoid roads with fast or congested traffic and stay on pavement and clearly marked footpaths. If you feel up to it, include at least one gradient, such as a low hill, in the route, depending on your level of fitness.

Start out slowly, with your shoulders relaxed and your head up. As you begin to warm up, gradually increase speed until you reach a comfortable, steady pace. Work on developing a relaxed walking style with broad strides, and swing your arms in time with your legs. Your breathing will become a little deeper and you will become warmer.

As you reach the end of your walk, gradually slow your pace down until your breathing returns to normal. Spread your walking sessions out across the week, with rest days in

Preparation and safety

Sneakers are fine for walking on dry, flat surfaces, but on hilly, wet, or rough ground you need boots that provide good support and have deeply treaded soles for good grip. Wear thick socks for

warmth and to prevent blisters. In cold weather it's better to wear several thinner layers of clothing rather than just one thick garment.

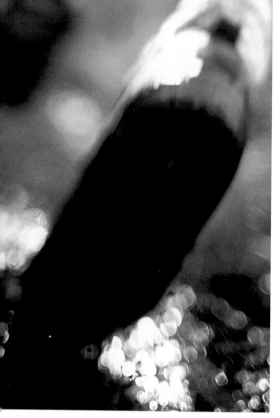

Walking boots come in a variety of materials. Synthetic materials are lighter, but leather offers better protection on rugged or difficult walks, so think about the terrain on which you will be walking.

When trying out boots or shoes, check that your ankle doesn't rise up as you walk.

Your toes should not touch the end of your boots; make sure that you can wriggle them freely and there is room for thick socks.

CHOOSING THE BEST BOOTS
Take time to choose your walking boots, preferably in a store where you can get advice from specialists.

between. You will steadily move faster and find that you need more demanding walks as you progress.

Rambling and hiking

Countryside covered with a network of trails and footpaths offers a variety of rewards in the form of picturesque scenery, undisturbed nature, and peacefulness. Many trails are not easy; you should check the degree of difficulty first, perhaps with a local walking or hiking club, a park ranger, or tourist office. If you want to try very ambitious routes, get expert advice on how to outfit yourself and some training in mountain skills and map reading. Prepare for a long ramble with a series of shorter walks of increasing length.

When walking up or down a hill, you increase your workload and energy expenditure considerably, compared to walking on a flat area. Walking downhill uses the leg muscles opposite to those involved when walking uphill. Unaccustomed downhill walking may make you sore because it uses certain muscles as shock absorbers. If you are planning a hill-walking vacation, include rest days to allow muscles to recover.

For a day-long hike, wear a lightweight backpack that holds ample water, food, and snacks, a first-aid kit, a compass, and a map of the area where you will be hiking. Wear your backpack as high as possible to avoid back strain.

Always respect the rules of the countryside or those posted at a trailhead. Stay on the trail or right-of-way and don't venture into areas where "no trespassing" signs are posted. In farm country, close gates behind you and keep dogs on a leash near farm animals.

Check the weather forecast before venturing out and seek the advice of experienced local walkers about problem areas along your route. If the weather is uncertain, carry a lightweight weatherproof jacket. Always inform a responsible person about the route you are taking and your expected time of return.

PLANNING YOUR WALKING ROUTE

You can make walks more interesting and gain maximum fitness benefits from them for the whole family by planning your route in advance. A town walk could take in historic features, a park, or a river towpath, for example, to vary the physical demands and maintain interest en route. In most towns and cities, plaques draw attention to the former homes of famous people.

Country walks can be planned to include hills for a good workout. Woodlands and riverbanks offer varied terrain with interesting sights and sounds, particularly for younger children. Make sure that you follow the country code when walking.

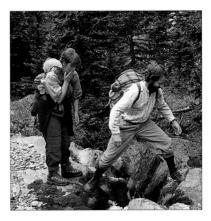

COUNTRY WALK
Climbing over rocky or difficult terrain gives the muscles of the upper body a workout. Walking up and down hills helps to strengthen muscles and bones, particularly of the legs and back.

Indoor treadmill walking

If it is dark, cold, icy, foggy, or extremely windy outside, treadmill walking is a suitable substitute for an outdoor walk. It is also a good way to plot your fitness progress because many modern treadmills can be programmed to emulate various terrains. This will help you achieve the best possible workout without braving the weather.

Walking tips

▶ *Wear loose, comfortable clothing appropriate to the weather, including headgear; 40 percent of body heat is lost from the head and neck.*

▶ *Always check the weather forecast before setting out.*

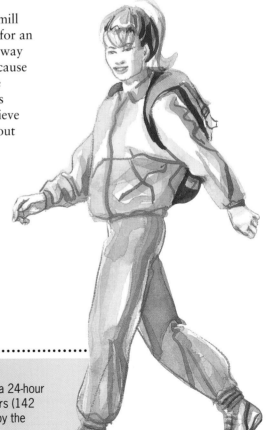

Fact file
The greatest distance walked in a 24-hour period so far is 228.93 kilometers (142 miles, 440 yards), a record set by the American Jose Castenada in Albuquerque, New Mexico, in 1976.

RUNNING

Running and jogging are excellent ways of strengthening the heart and lungs. The only difference between them is one of pace: jogging is done at a slow to moderate pace, whereas running is faster—sometimes at speeds up to an all-out sprint.

Running and jogging can be done alone or with a friend; runs can be easy or hard, competitive or friendly. You can run at any time of the day or night, anywhere you happen to be, and for however long you want.

Preparation and safety

When running on hard surfaces, such as pavement, wear shoes with cushioned soles that will reduce the impact on the knee and ankle joints. At night it is safer to run in groups and to stick to lighted streets, keeping away from dark alleys and subways. It is a good idea also to inform someone of your route details and expected time of return. Don't run while listening to a personal stereo; you will not be able to hear approaching cars. Never run when suffering from a viral illness or fever. Once you are completely recovered, start gently and build up your speed and distance very gradually.

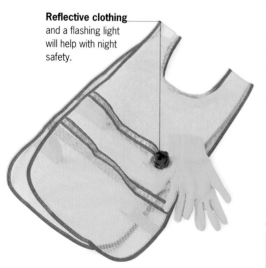

Reflective clothing and a flashing light will help with night safety.

NIGHTTIME SAFETY
On busy roads, make sure you can be seen by wearing light-colored or reflective clothing and running facing traffic.

Whereas sprinting is an anaerobic activity that requires a great deal of power output from the muscles, jogging and other forms of long-distance running are aerobic activities that call for muscular endurance. Because running is a high-impact activity, it can help maintain or increase bone density and thus lower the risk of osteoporosis. However, it does place a lot of stress on joints.

Getting started

To start running, all you need is a little enthusiasm and a comfortable pair of running shoes. You may also want to apply some petroleum jelly to parts of the body that rub against clothing, such as the top of the legs and arms. For women a well-fitted sports bra is essential. Wear loose, nonrestrictive clothing; in summer shorts and a T-shirt are fine. In winter a sweat suit or pair of thermal tights, a long-sleeved thermal top, and a windproof jacket are ideal. In very cold weather you should wear gloves and a hooded jacket or hat because a lot of body heat is lost through the hands and head.

Running tips

▶ *Keep your body straight, not leaning back or swaying from side to side.*

▶ *Swing your arms in a relaxed manner, keeping them close to the body.*

▶ *Try to keep steps light and spring so that the ankles and the calf and thigh muscles share the work equally.*

▶ *Avoid overstriding and high back kicks.*

Fact file
The fastest runners—100-meter sprinters—can achieve speeds above 43 km/h (27 mph). But such speeds are not sustainable for long. The average speed of runners who do a mile is around 26 km/h (16 mph).

Running requires no special equipment, apart from well-cushioned shoes. It provides good stamina- and bone-building exercise but can place excess stress on the joints.

As with all exercise you must start by warming up. Set off walking briskly and swinging your arms vigorously, then gradually break into a slow jog. Your level of fitness will determine when you are ready to step up the pace. Listen to your body. Although your breathing will be heavier than normal, you should not be so out of breath that you can't talk. Run at a pace at which you can hold a conversation. If you are getting too breathless to talk,

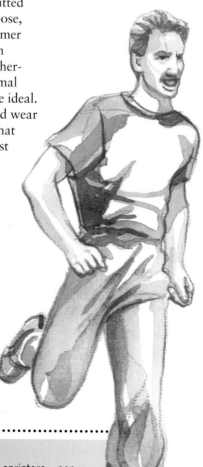

DIFFERENT FORMS OF RUNNING

Whether you choose fun runs, marathons, or track events, your technique will be of utmost importance. Fun runs allow each runner to complete the course at his or her own pace and generally require stamina rather than speed. Events on an athletic track, particularly sprints and field events, require the muscle power to produce short bursts of high speed. Such events as middle- and long-distance running demand a mixture of the speed and stamina needed to run for long periods at a more moderate pace.

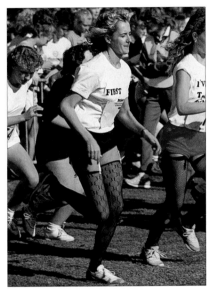

FUN RUNS
Designed to allow everyone to enjoy the pleasure of running, fun runs are highly sociable and mainly non-competitive. People of many ages can run together at a pace suitable to all.

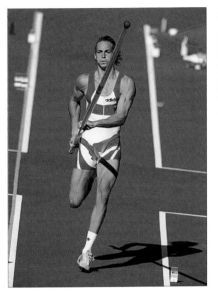

FIELD EVENTS
Many track events, such as the long jump, triple jump, and pole vault, require sprinting power. Athletes must develop strong leg and gluteal muscles in order to generate rapid acceleration.

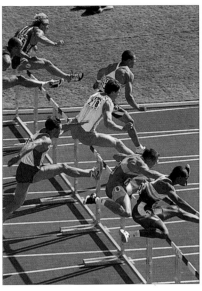

HURDLES
A hurdler requires several forms of fitness. Hurdling incorporates sprinting speed with jumping ability; such athletes must have good timing and speed, as well as accuracy and agility.

slow down or walk until you have recovered, then set off again.

As you run, put your heel down first and roll through to your toes. Try to stay relaxed, especially through the shoulders, and avoid using more effort than necessary. Sprinters have to lift their knees high to gain extra power, but joggers and distance runners should aim for lower and smaller steps.

At the end of each session you must cool down. Slow down gradually, finishing with a slow jog or brisk walk, until your heart rate and breathing return to more normal levels. While your muscles are still warm, do your stretches, concentrating in particular on the calves, quadriceps, hamstrings, abductors, and hip flexors.

Cross-country running

If you feel that jogging is not taxing enough, cross-country running may be the answer. You can make the course as difficult as you want and also set the speed to suit your current level of fitness and exercise goals. Cross-country running requires great stamina and strength because the various forms of terrain place different demands on the body.

When you plan your cross-country route, try to include grass, woodland, some pavement, and if possible, a sandy area. Also aim to vary the gradients you run on to include both hills and level surfaces. A 1-mile run on a firm, level surface is much easier than a mile run over hills and dunes, so don't overdo it at first. Gradually extend the distance that you cover

and/or the speed at which you are running until you feel you are getting a full workout.

To make cross-country running a mental challenge as well as a test of stamina and strength, many people take up orienteering, in which runners use maps to find their way between fixed control points. In addition to aerobic fitness and muscular strength, orienteering requires good navigational and tactical skills to find the quickest route between the control points.

Orienteering courses range from 1 km (just over half a mile) to about 16 km (10 miles) and vary in difficulty, depending on the age and experience of those taking part. There are courses for all ages, from children to the elderly.

SWIMMING

Swimming is very popular with all age groups and provides an all-round fitness workout. It improves the condition of the heart and lungs and works both upper and lower body muscles. Regular swimming will help to maintain strength, stamina, and flexibility, especially in the shoulders. Good swimming ability is also an important safety requirement for other water sports. Swimming can be informal, done just for recreation and fitness, or involve serious training and competition. Swim clubs generally cater to all age groups, often with opportunities for the more senior swimmers to become involved in coaching or the running of the club.

Preparation and safety

Take great care when swimming in open water. Sudden changes in temperature in lakes and rivers, particularly below the surface or in the shadow of trees, can cause debilitating and potentially fatal muscle cramps. Tides and currents can also cause problems, even for the most experienced swimmers. Seemingly calm stretches of water can have dangerously strong currents beneath the surface. Don't swim alone in unfamiliar water and never swim after drinking alcohol or within an hour of eating a large meal.

Adjustable straps will ensure a watertight fit.

Getting started

The main item needed is a swimsuit or swimming trunks. Learners may find buoyancy aids, such as armbands and floats, useful until they feel confident in the water. A swimming cap is advisable if you have long hair; goggles and a nose clip are helpful if you are sensitive to chlorinated water or the salt water of the sea; and ear plugs may be advisable for anyone who is prone to ear infections.

Most operators of swimming pools offer lessons for improving technique and set aside times during the week for people who wish to swim laps. There are also many advantages to

Swimming requires little equipment and therefore minimal expense. It boosts strength, suppleness and stamina, and the water's buoyancy aids the disabled and those with joint disorders.

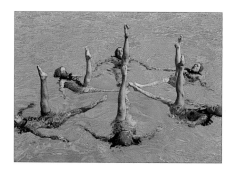

SYNCHRONIZED SWIMMING
Advanced swimmers who prefer a different challenge from speed or distance swimming may enjoy synchronized swimming. Somewhat like dancing, synchronized swimming demands a great deal of strength, stamina, and flexibility, coupled with control, gracefulness, and a sense of timing.

training with a swim club, in addition to the fun of competition. Each session is set for you by the coach, who will help you improve your stroke and breathing techniques. Strong swimmers can enroll in a lifesaving course, in which they

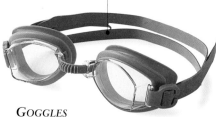

GOGGLES
Goggles help to protect your eyes from the irritation of chlorine or salt water and allow you to see more clearly when swimming. They should be watertight and fit snugly around the eyes and nose.

Swimming tips

▶ *Keep your body as streamlined (stretched out) as possible to reduce water resistance.*

▶ *Breathe rhythmically while swimming and tailor your stroke to make breathing easier.*

▶ *If you feel tired, tread water or turn over onto your back and float until you feel ready to continue swimming. The body is naturally buoyant.*

▶ *Swim with a partner so that you can encourage each other.*

Fact file
Swimming was recorded as far back as 36 B.C. in Japan, yet three competition strokes, front and back crawl and butterfly, are 20th-century inventions. The fourth, breast stroke, dates from the 16th century.

will not only learn how to do water rescues but also master resuscitation techniques while improving their swimming skills as well.

Pool-based sports

Many swimming techniques can be used to play pool-based sports, such as octopush and water polo.

Octopush is a form of underwater hockey; it provides particularly good stamina and muscle-building exercise and is great fun as well.

Water polo, which was developed in the mid-1800s, has grown so much in popularity that it is now an Olympic event. It is described as being a cross between swimming and football. Nets are set at either end of the pool, and each team tries to score goals in the opposition's net by passing the ball or dribbling it— pushing the ball ahead—while swimming toward the goal. Strong swimming skills, speed, and agility are necessary to play at most levels, but simpler versions of the game can be played in shallow water with the water acting as a cushion against dives for the ball.

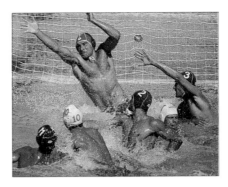

WATER POLO
A physically demanding sport, water polo requires constant activity—treading water, swimming, and throwing the ball.

ROWING AND PADDLING

In the sport of rowing, there are two or more participants, each person handling one oar. For sculling, one rower uses two smaller oars.

Paddling involves the use of a special kind of rowing device called a paddle. It has a blade at both ends for kayaking or at one end only for canoeing. Kayaks and canoes that are maneuvered by one person require individual skill and effort; when paddled by two or more people, they call for teamwork.

Rowing is regarded by many as a complete exercise. It utilizes most of the major muscles of the body and can tax them at varying intensities, offering both aerobic and anaerobic work. Paddling requires good upper body strength, while rowing makes demands on both the leg muscles and the upper body.

Getting started

Paddling and rowing are taught at special clubs and outdoor recreation centers and are favorite competitive sports at many universities. As with all water sports, it is important that you be a competent swimmer and have good knowledge of water safety before you go out in a boat.

An instructor will teach you skills you need to handle a particular craft and the rules and dangers specific to the waterways you will be using. A kayak, which is a mostly enclosed craft, can overturn and trap the inexperienced paddler; the first thing you will be taught is the Eskimo roll—an intentional overturning and righting of the kayak—so that you can right your craft in the event of capsize. You will then be ready to practice the other basic techniques.

Until you have become fairly proficient and are able to right your craft or swim it ashore in the event of a capsizing, you should never row or paddle alone on unfamiliar water.

> Rowing and paddling require some financial outlay for club fees and rental or purchase of equipment. They are good for building stamina and upper body strength and endurance.

Rowing machines

Machines that mimic rowing on water have made the sport more widely accessible. The action is non-weight-bearing and the intensity level easily adaptable, so it is suitable for people of all ages and fitness levels, except those with back disorders.

Preparation and safety

Bad rowing technique can result in chronic lower back disorders. Correct technique involves keeping a straight back. When you pull back on the oars, make the effort come from your legs and arms, not your back. When paddling, keep a smooth steady stroke and twist your upper body from the hips.

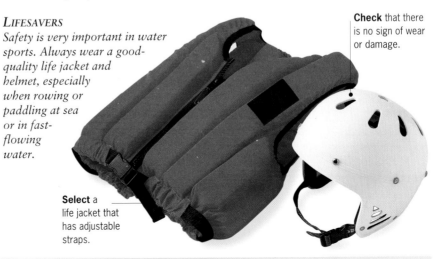

LIFESAVERS
Safety is very important in water sports. Always wear a good-quality life jacket and helmet, especially when rowing or paddling at sea or in fast-flowing water.

Check that there is no sign of wear or damage.

Select a life jacket that has adjustable straps.

CYCLING

Cycling is an excellent activity for strengthening your heart and lungs, relieving stress, and increasing muscular strength and endurance. It is also good for building anaerobic fitness and tolerance to lactic acid (see page 33) because the large leg muscles produce excess amounts of this waste product during cycling.

Cycling is an inexpensive and pollution-free means of transport. Riding a bicycle to and from work or school integrates exercise into everyday activities, while cycling during leisure time is a great way to explore the countryside. With the growing interest in cycling in recent years, competitive events, clubs, and travel tours have increased and cater to almost everyone, from the serious rider to the occasional cyclist.

Many bicycle clubs exist throughout North America. Some are aimed at cyclists who want to ride with a group and set themselves challenges but do not want to race. Others cater to competitive road-race, track, and time-trial cyclists. Mountain bike clubs are for those who want to explore the countryside or orienteer

on a bike or who like to race off-road. These clubs welcome all ages and experience levels, and some also have children's divisions. Many local and national parks allow mountain biking on specified trails. And some ski resorts operate their lifts in summer so that bikers can get to the top of a mountain and ride down.

Getting started

An important consideration in choosing a bike is getting the right size. If a bicycle is the wrong size or is incorrectly adjusted, you will have an uncomfortable ride and are at greater risk for injury. It is especially dangerous for children to ride a bike that is too large for them because they will not be able to control it properly. As a general guide, the stand-over height of the bicycle—the distance between the crossbar and the top of the rider's inside leg when straddling the bike—should be at least 7 to 8 cm (about 3 in). The seat, pedals, and handlebars must also be adjusted to the individual.

Most stores adjust the bicycle when it is purchased and advise on

Cycling provides good aerobic and muscle-building exercise but requires an initial financial outlay and a commitment to training to ensure safe and problem-free riding.

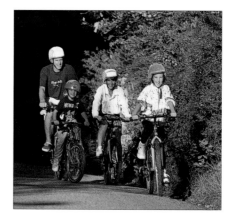

FAMILY OUTINGS
Cycling can be a great way to enjoy family outings. Children should always be taught road safety and cycling proficiency before riding on the roads.

suitable clothing and the correct helmet. Padded cycle shorts improve comfort, and a close-fitting cycle jersey reduces wind resistance and prevents a buildup of moisture.

A common mistake that beginners make is incorrect use of gears. Using too high a gear causes leg fatigue very quickly. Choose a gear that allows you to turn the pedals smoothly without straining too much—a low gear for cycling uphill and a higher gear for downhill.

A warm-up is always necessary. You should start out slowly, then gradually increase the workload by pedaling faster or using a higher gear. Incorporate a gradual cooldown at the end of each session.

On-road cycling

An all-purpose tourer is a good investment for someone who wishes to use cycling to explore the countryside or to commute to work. These bicycles are generally light and have several gears in order to cope with hills and changing traffic speeds. They also have mudguards,

---

Preparation and safety

It is important to maintain your equipment. Carrying a small tool kit is recommended because punctures and minor wheel damage are common, especially on poorly maintained roads and rough terrain. Make sure you can be clearly seen by other road users at all times. In many regions it is illegal to cycle at night without a white light in front and a red light at the rear.

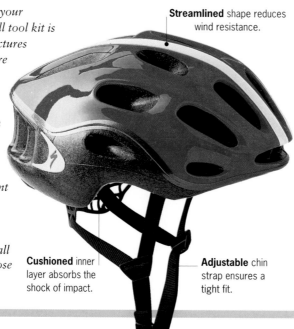

Streamlined shape reduces wind resistance.

Cushioned inner layer absorbs the shock of impact.

Adjustable chin strap ensures a tight fit.

CYCLING HELMET
A safety helmet is vital for all cyclists, but particularly those who cycle in traffic or over rough ground.

brakes, which are essential for safety in traffic. Some racing bicycles have curved handlebars but it is important to hold the top of these when cycling on busy roads, or to choose a bicycle with straight handlebars. Bending to hold the curved bars can produce excessive tension in the neck and shoulders, cramp the abdomen, and impair breathing. Crouching over the bicycle can also be dangerous on the road as it impairs your field of vision, so curved handlebars should be used only for racing or off-road cycling where there is little danger of traffic accidents.

Before you cycle on the road, make sure you know the highway code and that you have reached a good degree of cycling proficiency. Wear bright-coloured, reflective or fluorescent strips or clothing and ensure your lights are in good working order.

Off-road cycling

For more adventurous cycling, off-road and exploring hard-to-get-to places, a mountain bike is the better option. These have wide tyres to grip both soft and hard surfaces, and the frames are light but also very strong to withstand the excessive stress and strain put on them. Mountain bikes are designed with sport in mind, so they do not usually have luggage carriers or mudguards like touring cycles, as these would make them heavier and slower. They have very low gears so that the cyclist can climb steep inclines, and high gears to make it easier to descend.

Off-road cycling requires more upper body strength and greater balance than road cycling, but the rewards are a traffic-free environment and access to places that are unattainable by car.

A good way to start off-road riding is to put the bike in the car and take it to a place with some fairly level off-road trails. Always check beforehand that you are not cycling on private or restricted land. When you start cycling off-road do not plan to cover the same distance that you would on roads as you will be travelling much slower for the same amount of effort.

Cycling tips

▶ *Always carry a basic tool kit, comprising tyre levers, puncture repair kit (adhesive, sandpaper and patches) and a spare inner tube, if possible.*

▶ *Make sure that your lights and reflectors are clean and working.*

▶ *Wear a good-quality smog mask in heavy traffic.*

Fact file

The modern pedal bicycle was invented in Scotland in 1840 and has developed over 150 years into the many specialist varieties of racing, mountain and touring bikes popular today.

TYPES OF CYCLE

When choosing a bicycle, bear in mind the type of cycling you will want to do and the road conditions or terrain you will be facing. For example, a racing bicycle may not be suitable for riding along pot-holed country roads. Specialist bicycle shops offer information on choosing the most suitable bicycle.

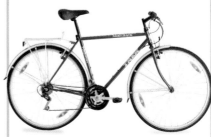

ALL-PURPOSE TOURER
A sturdy bicycle, the traditional tourer is favoured for its versatility and reliability.

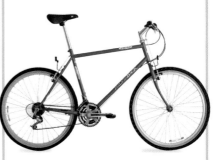

MOUNTAIN BIKE
Cycling over rugged terrain demands a strong, durable frame and sturdy tyres.

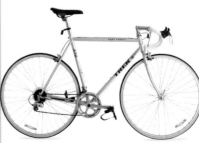

RACING BIKE
The light frame and drop handlebars make the racing bike ideal for speed. The position of the handlebars curves your body into a streamlined shape.

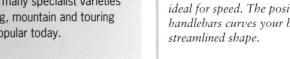

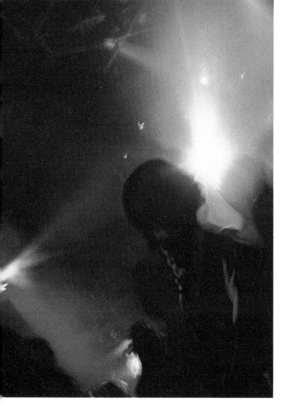

Dancing

Dancing, from which there are hundreds of styles to choose, is an enjoyable and sociable way of improving heart and lung fitness and toning the body. Many professional sports people include some form of dance in their training.

JAZZ AND TAP

Jazz and tap dancing are more energetic than many other forms of dance and are excellent for toning and strengthening the legs and feet. Once the basic steps have been learned, they can be combined in any way the dancer wishes. This means that you can tailor your workout to suit your own needs.

Getting started
It is almost impossible to learn jazz or tap without joining a class. Once you have mastered the basics, you

Jazz and tap dancing help develop all-round fitness, though some people may find them physically too demanding. Many of the steps take time to learn and can require natural ability.

can choose whether to remain in the class environment or not. Jazz and tap are not especially social forms of dance; it may be difficult to find fellow dancers without taking a class. Many classes enter competitions and put on special performances to keep their members motivated and allow them to show off their skills.

LINE DANCING

Line dancing, which originated in the midwestern and southern states, has quickly become one of the most popular forms of contemporary dancing. You don't need a partner for line dancing because, as its name suggests, the dances are performed in lines, or rows, of dancers.

Line dancing is a very sociable activity because you are dancing the same steps at the same time with dozens of people rather than alone or as a couple. Most line dances have simple step patterns that are easy to learn and are not too physically taxing. Once you have mastered the basic steps, you will soon be able to line dance to almost any popular song you hear.

Physically, line dancing has an effect similar to that of a low-impact aerobics class, which makes it a good form of cardiovascular exercise. It

consists mostly of step work—in fact, the hands are often held still by keeping the thumbs in the pockets—so line dancing is generally of most

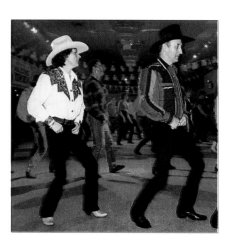

LINE DANCING
Fun and highly sociable, line dancing has become a very popular dance form with all age groups.

Line dancing is inexpensive, easy to learn, and highly sociable. It offers gentle aerobic exercise without being too demanding, but it will not provide all-round physical fitness.

benefit to the lower body. For all-round fitness you will have to find an additional activity that works the upper body.

Getting started
It is easiest to begin line dancing by enrolling in a class or joining in at a club or bar that features it. Because of the growing popularity of line dancing, most towns have a place that offers lessons or holds dancing evenings and will welcome newcomers. You can practice the dances alone or with a partner, but the real enjoyment comes from dancing in step with a large group.

BALLROOM

Ballroom dancing not only is a good way to exercise but also helps develop coordination and good posture. Ballroom is made up mainly of two disciplines, modern and Latin, and can range from fast, energetic dancing, to slower, graceful styles. The basics are fairly easy to learn because all dances are based on simple steps set to a specific rhythm.

An evening spent ballroom dancing, particularly in a class, provides a complete exercise session, with warm-up and cool-down routines and, as dancing progresses, a full aerobic workout.

Dancing greatly improves suppleness and stamina, especially in the faster forms, such as jive. For a beginner, however, the exercise is a less intense workout because the emphasis is placed on learning position and posture. As you become more familiar with the dances, you can concentrate more on the fitness elements. Sports that involve fluid movements, such as cycling and swimming, combine well with dance.

OTHER DANCES

There are many types of popular dance offered. Classes for special forms—from salsa, flamenco, and lambada to disco and even square dancing—can be found in most areas. These are all excellent ways of improving coordination and strength and for building up cardiovascular fitness. Most classes cater to dancers at all levels, but don't underestimate the demands of dance; make sure you warm up well before a session and stretch before and after. Some more advanced dance classes incorporate ballet training to improve suppleness, posture, and muscular strength.

Getting started

Ballroom dance classes are held in community halls and private dance studios, and there are social events, such as tea dances, that include some tuition. You can learn as one of a group or opt for one-on-one instruction. Most schools welcome new dancers of every level, but it may be worthwhile observing a class first to see if it will be of benefit to you, depending on your level of experience. Individual instruction is more expensive but enables you to learn the basics more quickly.

Many people enjoy the chance to dress up that ballroom dancing affords, but casual clothes are acceptable at most dance schools. The most suitable are loose pants for men and a flowing skirt for women. Ballroom dancing provides an exercise routine for people of all ages and fitness levels.

Ballroom dancing requires a commitment to learn and may take many years to master the fine points. It provides all-round exercise, relaxation, and a strong social element.

Preparation and safety

Lighter and more flexible than ordinary shoes, dance shoes have brushed suede soles and nonskid heels for a good floor grip. You can adapt ordinary shoes by fitting them with special stick-on soles.

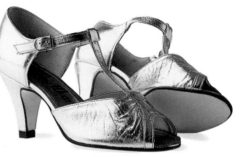

DANCING FEET
It is important to wear shoes for dancing that are well fitted and comfortable and have soles that glide smoothly.

Dancing tips

▶ *Wear loose, comfortable clothing that does not restrict your movements.*

▶ *Warm up beforehand and cool down and stretch thoroughly afterward.*

▶ *Move your legs freely from the hips and keep a fluid action in the knees.*

▶ *Don't forget to use your arms, hands, torso, and head too.*

Fact file
Ballroom dancing requires music played at a strict tempo by dance bands. For example, the tango and samba are danced in 2/4 time; the waltz is in 3/4 time; and the foxtrot, jive, and quickstep are in 4/4 time.

Team Sports

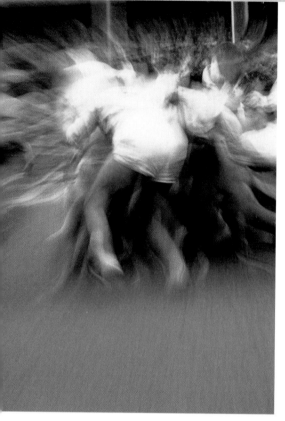

Team sports are especially suitable for anyone who enjoys the camaraderie of a closely knit group of like-minded people. Also, the encouragement and support of other team members can help motivate a person to keep fit.

RUGBY

There are two main forms of rugby—union and league. Both involve running, passing the ball, and tackling. Rugby union includes more set-piece moves, which make the game more tactical and less flowing in nature. Rugby league has simpler rules and fewer set pieces, so that running and passing represent a larger proportion of the game and there are fewer stoppages.

Getting started

Many people play rugby at school and then lose touch with the game when they leave. Getting back into the sport can be difficult because you have to prepare yourself physically and reacquire the skills that are needed. For these reasons it is necessary to start by joining an established rugby club. Rugby was traditionally a male-only sport, but today there are many women's teams. The game is intensely physical, demanding a high degree of upper body strength. It also requires speed and agility for sprinting and quick directional changes, coupled with strength in the legs, arms, and shoulders for tackling and scrums (in which both sides scramble to take possession of the ball when it is tossed up).

> Rugby and American football are ideal for people who enjoy competition, camaraderie, and rough physical contact. For optimum enjoyment and safety, you need stamina and strength.

Touch football

Developed as an alternative to the rough physical contact of traditional football, touch football has become especially popular with teams for children and women. Instead of tackling, players have to touch the opposing player who is carrying the ball.

Rugby tips

▶ *Resistance training, either with free weights or machines, is very important for building both strength and muscle bulk.*

▶ *An aerobic training program based on running will help delay the onset of fatigue.*

Fact file

Rugby was invented during a soccer match at its namesake school in England in 1823, when William Webb Ellis picked up the ball and ran with it.

THE DEMANDS OF TEAM BALL GAMES

Team ball games are mainly multiple sprint sports, in which the individual is alternately sprinting, jogging, walking, or standing still. The muscular demands of these actions are interspersed with the power and coordination required to catch, strike, throw, or kick the ball. Depending on which game you are playing, your position on the field, and the level at which the game is being played, varying degrees of fitness and combinations of the components of fitness (see page 52) are needed. Most clubs cater to a range of skill and fitness levels by having two or more teams of different standards.

SOCCER

Soccer can be played outdoors on a soccer field with 11 players per team, on a smaller indoor court with 5 or 6 players to a side, or as an informal - kick-around in the local park. The fitness demands depend on the level of playing and the player's position.

Getting started

The game can be enjoyed by people with any level of skill, but it is best played with others of similar ability. One approach is to encourage friends to join you for sessions at a local sports field or any suitable open ground. You can also set up a company team and play other firms in your area. The basic skills of the game are relatively easy to learn and quickly improve with practice.

Eleven-a-side soccer played on a full-sized field involves intermittent bouts of activity with rest breaks between sprints. Five-a-side and six-a-side games are much more energetic and afford few opportunities to rest; therefore, players need excellent stamina and muscular endurance if they are to last the full game.

A lack of stamina will reduce your playing ability because fatigue will set in earlier and affect your ball control and speed. The sudden changes in speed and direction involved in the game also put players at increased risk for joint and muscular injuries.

You can guard against injury by regularly doing exercises for strength and flexibility. A good way to prepare for the physical stress of the game is to do circuit training (see page 125), incorporating exercises that concentrate particularly on the running, jumping, twisting, and turning elements of the game.

Soccer is an inexpensive game that can be enjoyed at all skill levels. It offers all-round exercise, but for safety you should aim to get reasonably fit before playing.

Soccer tips

▶ *To reduce the risk of injury, especially after not playing for a long time, players must build muscle strength and develop cardiovascular fitness with regular aerobic activities.*

▶ *Whether passing, shooting, heading, or tackling, keep your eye on the ball until the moment you play it.*

Fact file
Modern soccer was organized in England in the early 19th century, but a form of the game was played by the ancient Greeks, Romans, Chinese, and Egyptians.

Preparation and safety

Soccer or rugby shoes are best for playing on grass, while cross trainers are more suitable for playing indoors or on asphalt. Soccer is not usually considered a dangerous sport, although knee and ankle injuries are common. Regular fitness training can help reduce this risk. Rugby and football, however, are potentially dangerous contact sports that demand high levels of fitness, strength, and flexibility at all levels of the game.

Before you start to play, train well to meet the physical demands of the sport.

PLAYING SAFE
Most players recommend using some protective equipment, such as gum shields in rugby and shin pads in soccer.

SOCCER OPTIONS

If you would like to get involved in playing soccer but do not feel you have the particular skills needed to be a striker, midfield player, or defender, all is not lost. There are two other important roles you could play: goalkeeper or referee. The first, one of the most important positions on a team, calls for the ability to catch, throw, and kick the ball, as well as to tackle. The second can give you a full workout as you run to keep track of the game but it does not demand the skills of a team player.

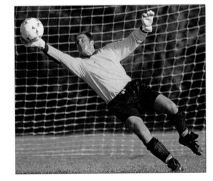

GOAL!
The position of goalkeeper requires agility and good hand-eye coordination but not the cardiovascular demands of the other positions.

BASKETBALL AND NETBALL

Basketball and netball are team games played on outdoor or indoor courts. Both are relatively simple and and can be enjoyed by beginners with little initial training. Basketball is played at most high schools and colleges and in local associations. Netball, more popular in the United Kingdom and Europe than North America, is not played competitively in a number of states. Both games involve frequent changes of speed and direction, bending, and jumping, and require a good level of aerobic fitness, as well as coordination, suppleness, balance, and ball skills.

Each team defends a hoop or basket affixed to a post with a backboard at one end of the court and scores by shooting the ball through the opposing team's hoop or basket at the other end.

One main difference between the two games is the way the ball is moved around the court. In netball, the ball is thrown from one player to another, and the player holding the ball must keep one foot in place and pass the ball to another player within three seconds. In basketball, players also throw or pass the ball to each other, but a player can also run with it—as long as he or she constantly bounces, or dribbles, it while running.

Getting started

You need relatively strong, supple joints to cope with the frequent changes of direction, jumping, and twisting during a game. A degree of strength in the arms and hands is also necessary for catching and throwing the ball. It is helpful to strengthen the muscles through regular resistance and stretching exercises and to warm up well before playing a game.

Netball and basketball tips

▶ *Keep your steps loose and springy, your knees slightly flexed, and your feet apart, especially as you land after jumping.*

▶ *In netball only designated players can shoot for the net, or hoop, but in basketball any player can score.*

▶ *An important skill in basketball is dribbling, which can be practiced alone.*

Netball and basketball are inexpensive to play and, apart from the ball and baskets, require only sport shorts or skirts, a top, and good training shoes. Both games aid all-round fitness.

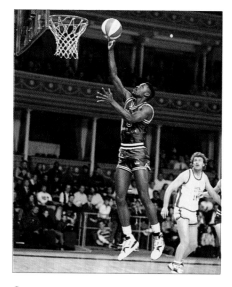

SPRING POWER
Scoring in basketball or netball requires leg strength to gain extra height and supple wrists and fingers for shooting.

It is also useful to spend time practicing the techniques of the game, such as passing, shooting, and dribbling, as this will enhance both your skills and your physical fitness.

To get the most out of basketball and netball, you should build up a basic level of fitness before you begin to play competitively. Strength, stamina, and agility are all important. During a game a player can run up to 5 kilometers (3 miles), usually in short, fast bursts of sprinting, and the rest of the time must keep moving to guard the opposing players.

Fact file

Modern basketball was invented by a Canadian, James Naismith, in 1891, but the Olmecs of Mexico played a similar game more than 1,200 years ago. Netball was also developed in the United States as a women's version of basketball but first gained popularity in Great Britain.

VOLLEYBALL

Volleyball was developed in 1895 by William Morgan, an American physical education instructor, as a simple sport that people of all fitness levels could play. Originally it consisted of an inflated bladder that was batted over a piece of rope. Today it is a popular six-a-side sport played indoors and out over a net.

Getting started
Simple to set up, volleyball requires minimal equipment and can be played almost anywhere and with as few as two players. There are not many rules to learn, so beginners quickly pick up the basics. It is best to join a team in order to learn the correct skills and develop a sense of team-work and tactical play.

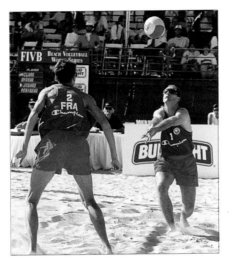

BEACH VOLLEYBALL
Volleyball played on a sand court or beach has become extremely popular because dives are cushioned by the sand.

Volleyball is a simple and enjoyable game for all skill levels. It does little to enhance stamina, however, and players need a degree of suppleness and strength to avoid injury.

Preparation and safety

It is a common mistake to think that volleyball requires little preparation. The stop-start nature of the game means there is a risk of joint and muscle injuries unless players do a thorough warm-up first. Using the correct arm position to play the ball also helps to prevent injury. It is important to use the right type of ball; avoid molded rubber balls, which can be painful on the arms and may discourage beginners.

FIELD HOCKEY

Field hockey can be played indoors or out with teams of 5 or 11 players. It is a fast game, involving steady running interspersed with sudden bursts of speed and rapid changes of direction that strengthen the lower body muscles. Upper body muscles are also strengthened by the constant use of the stick when dribbling,
passing, tackling, and shooting, while the constant, steady running provides an excellent cardio-vascular workout.

Preparation and safety

Field hockey is a fast game, and because it involves sticks and a small hard ball, it can be a dangerous one. Players should wear shin guards and knuckle and hand protectors. Because the ball is not always at ground level, many players also wear gum shields. Goalkeepers are well protected with large leg pads, kickers— metal foot protection—gloves, body padding, headgear, a face mask, and arm protectors. Sticks should be free of splinters and rough edges, which might make play dangerous, and must never be lifted above shoulder height during play. Players are advised not to wear jewelry.

Getting started
Hockey requires agility, stamina, and good hand-eye coordination. As with all team sports, it is necessary not only to join a team but also to commit to attending all regular training sessions, as well as the matches. To play well, it it essential to develop stick skills and team-playing ability; proficiency usually comes with lots of practice.

Fact file
A game like hockey was played in Greece around 2500 B.C. Modern hockey dates from 1875, when the English Hockey Association was founded.

Hockey requires only minimal equipment, but regular training sessions are necessary to maintain fitness and skills if players are to get the most from the game.

Hockey tips

► *To push the ball, hold your hands well apart along the stick and move the head of the stick in a steady sweeping movement.*

► *Never kick the ball—it is a foul in hockey except when the goalie does it. The only permissible way to move the ball is with the stick.*

CRICKET

Cricket differs from other games in the range of skills that players bring to it. Spin and fast bowling, fielding, and batting all require excellent hand-eye coordination. The various positions also demand different types of fitness. When fielding, quick reactions and flexibility are important. Medium and fast bowlers are constantly walking, running, and bowling the ball. As they tire, their bowling tends to become less accurate, so all-round muscular strength and endurance are required. Batsmen need upper body power to hit the ball with force and accuracy, as well as strength and flexibility for sprinting between the wickets.

Getting started

Cricket is an unusual sport in that matches can last many hours and—at the top class level—as long as several days. Most amateur cricketers play "limited over" matches, in which a limit is set on the number of balls that each side faces. Games like pairs and eight-a-side cricket, which are designed to hone skills, can be much shorter and also make

exciting competitions for all ages. Variations of the game are sometimes played indoors at sports centers, mainly to provide off-season training. Cricket involves skills that are acquired and honed mainly through constant training.

Because cricket can involve long periods of inactivity interspersed with sudden bursts of intense activity, the chances of injury are great. The muscles and joints can quickly become cold—especially at the start and end of the season, when the weather can be chilly. Also, when a player has to burst into action, the chances of incurring sprains and strains increase.

To avoid injury and enjoy the sport to the fullest, players must develop a high degree of cardiovascular fitness,

Cricket is a skilled game that requires a major commitment to be played competitively. To avoid injury and gain the most benefit, it is important to get fit before you play.

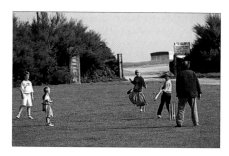

FAMILY CRICKET
The basic rules of cricket can be modified to create a variety of simple games that are suitable for the whole family to play.

flexibility, and stamina. They should also try to maintain and improve their fitness during the off-season and between matches to reduce their risk of injury. In particular, cricketers should work on muscular strength and endurance by doing resistance training, and on cardiovascular endurance with such aerobic activities as jogging. They should also work on general flexibility and mobility of the lower back and shoulders. As the playing season approaches, cricketers should consider including sprint drills in their program. A specially tailored system of circuit training that includes exercises to strengthen the muscles and joints most at risk in cricket can be particularly beneficial.

Preparation and safety

In cricket a hard ball is propelled at high speed, so there is a risk of serious injury, especially when a player is batting or keeping wicket. Gloves, leg pads, and a cricket box for men to protect the genitals are vital; for serious players a helmet with temple guards is also advisable.

Regular players usually prefer to use their own bat and gloves.

Cricket tips

▶ *When batting, stand with your feet a bat's width apart and your weight evenly distributed on both feet.*

▶ *Keep your eyes level and head fully turned toward the bowler; your shoulders should be in line and pointing down the wicket.*

▶ *Make use of the time between overs and any other delays in play to stretch your arm and leg muscles.*

Fact file
The first county cricket match was played in England in 1719, but a similar game was known as far back as the 16th century. Early batsmen defended either a tree stump or a wicket gate.

BASEBALL AND SOFTBALL

Baseball and softball are similar games that originated in the United States. The teams are made up of nine players, each side alternately batting and fielding (the teams change sides when the one at bat has acquired three outs). The aim is to hit the ball thrown by the pitcher and run around a diamond made up of three bases and home plate; a run is scored when a batter reaches home plate. This can be done in stages, but if a batter gets around all bases in one hit, it is called a home run.

Long a favorite pastime in the United States, baseball is now played in many countries, including Japan and Italy. The game can be very fast, requiring physical stamina and

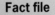

SOFTBALL
Softball can be enjoyed by people of any age and with less of the protective gear required in baseball.

fitness. It is best to build up fitness levels before taking up the sport. Stretching and warming up the muscles before playing are especially important to reduce the risk of injury.

Softball is a version of baseball in which the field of play is smaller and the ball is larger and lighter. Also, because the pitching action is underarm rather than overarm, the speed of the ball is reduced.

Softball is a social sport, and both men and women often take part in the same game. It is becoming increasingly popular in sports clubs and with many firms, which sponsor teams for playing after work hours.

Getting started
To prepare for the game, it helps to work on upper body strength—to aid in batting and throwing—and do aerobic and leg-strengthening

Baseball tips

▶ *Hold the bat at shoulder height and keep your eye on the approaching ball. Shoulders should be level and in line with the ball.*

▶ *As you hit, swing your upper body along with the bat and transfer your weight to the front foot to add force to the stroke.*

Baseball, softball, and rounders are fast and highly sociable games that can aid strength and suppleness when combined with a regular all-round exercise regimen.

exercises—to improve one's ability to get around the bases. "Batting cages" at sports centers allow players to practice batting skills.

Fact file
The origins of baseball are debated, but some attribute its modern invention to New Yorker Abner Doubleday in 1839.

ROUNDERS

Rounders, a game similar to softball, is played with a small hard ball and smaller bat. It is very popular in the United Kingdom, particularly with children. The game allows for both individual skills and teamwork. Rounders predates baseball by almost a century; the first reference to the game in England was in 1744.

Preparation and safety

The baseball is small and heavy and can cause injuries, so the catcher, who squats behind the batter and catches missed balls, must be protected with helmet, mask, chest and throat protectors, and leg guards. The batter wears a helmet, and players in the field use leather mitts to protect their hands when catching the ball.

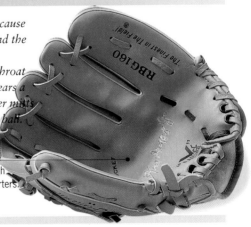

The catcher's mitt protects the player's hands from injury through impact with the ball at close quarters.

Racquet Sports

When played at a reasonable skill level against an opponent of equal ability, racquet sports provide excellent exercise. They tax all of the body's energy systems, requiring a combination of skill, stamina, strength, and coordination.

TENNIS

Tennis is a versatile, physically active sport that can be played indoors or out on grass, concrete, clay, or artificial turf courts. The game is played as either singles (two people) or doubles (four people), with doubles being less taxing than singles. Tennis has always included a strong social element, which attracts players who want to make new friends and socialize with old ones.

Tennis is an enjoyable and highly sociable game. Optimum health benefits can be experienced by evenly matched players who have reasonably good skills.

Getting started
Many clubs have both indoor and outdoor tennis courts and some also have "short tennis," played with softer balls on a smaller court with a lower net. This version is a good way for children to acquire the skills of the game.

If you have never played before, the best approach is to concentrate just on returning the ball over the net. Do not try to place powerful volleys, as these skills come only with experience. You can start off playing for only half an hour and gradually build up to playing for longer periods. When you feel fit enough, you can play full games and sets.

Tennis involves all the muscles and joints in the body, so warming up is crucial because your body will be stretched vigorously during a game. Tennis provides limited aerobic exercise, however, except at more advanced levels, because only skilled and evenly matched players can sustain rallies long enough to test their cardiovascular systems. For all-round fitness, do aerobic activities, such as brisk walking or jogging, as well.

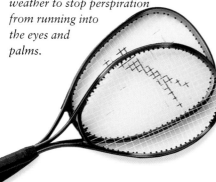

Tennis tips

▶ *Keep your wrist firm when striking the ball.*

▶ *Put your weight behind the racquet as you play the ball.*

Fact file
An early form of court tennis dates back to the 16th century, but lawn tennis is credited to Major Walter Clopton Wingfield, who introduced it at a party in Wales in 1873.

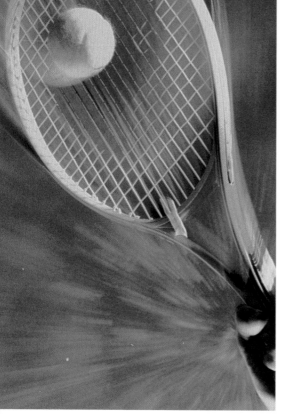

Preparation and safety

Clothing suitable for tennis and other racquet sports allows unrestricted movement, particularly of the arms. Sweat-absorbent wristbands and headbands are recommended in warm weather to stop perspiration from running into the eyes and palms.

CHOOSING A TENNIS RACQUET
Check that the racquet is evenly balanced, not weighted in the head or the handle, and make sure the grip feels comfortable in both size and shape.

SQUASH AND RACQUETBALL

Squash was developed at Harrow school in England around 1850 and was originally played with a softer ball. It was derived from rackets, an earlier sport from the Middle Ages that is thought to be the precursor of most racquet games. Squash is played in a four-walled court with a ceiling and springs beneath the floor. When struck, the ball must first hit the front wall but can then bounce off the four walls, which means that it is kept in play longer than is possible in most racquet sports. For this reason squash usually provides a thorough cardiovascular workout. The smallness of the court and the speed of the returns means that the game can be extremely fast.

Racquetball—another descendant of rackets—is similar to squash but is a more modern sport, having been developed in America in the 1950s

from a combination of court handball and paddleball. In this game the ball can be played off the ceiling as well as the walls. Racquetball can be played by two, four, or three players; this last version is called cutthroat.

Getting started

Both games are played in specially designed courts that can be found at most sports and health clubs. It is advisable to play a little to see if the game is for you before buying equipment; many courts have racquets for rent if you can't borrow one. The different colored spots on squash balls denote their speed and determine the degree of difficulty— the slower the ball, the harder the game. Both sports are very demanding and should be played only by people with good stamina.

Squash and racquetball are sociable games that are physically demanding and suitable only for the very fit. To play, one must pay rent for a court or for a membership in a health club.

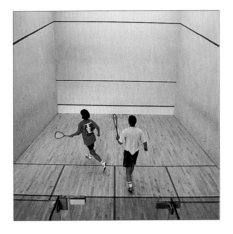

THE COURT
The lines around the walls of a squash court denote the areas into which the ball can be hit and remain in play.

BADMINTON

Badminton is played on a court with a high net. Although it is usually played indoors, it can also be played outdoors on a calm day. The players use a light, long-handled racquet to volley a shuttlecock, traditionally made of cork and feathers, which must not touch the ground during play. (The design of a shuttlecock keeps it in the air longer than would be the case with a ball.)

Badminton is usually played with two or four players on the court, although it is possible to proceed with three. It can be played at virtually any pace, from a leisurely knockabout one to a fiercely competitive and frenetic speed.

Getting started

While the most skilled players are very fast, it is possible for less experienced players and anyone just taking up the sport to have an enjoyable and energetic game. For this

reason badminton is an ideal game for people who have been inactive for a long time and are now planning to build up their fitness levels, as well as for those who are looking for more energetic exercise.

Badminton is an enjoyable and sociable game suitable for all ages, abilities, and fitness levels. It offers an all-round workout—even for beginners to the game.

Badminton tips

▶ *Stand on the balls of the feet with knees slightly bent to create a springy stance.*

▶ *Always return to a central position on the court between strokes to be prepared for the next one.*

Fact file
Modern badminton was developed at Badminton House, England, in the 1800s, but a similar game was played in China 2,000 years ago.

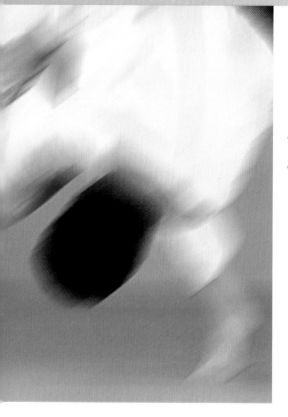

Eastern Exercise

Many forms of exercise that originated in India and the Orient have the ability to calm the mind and spirit and enhance self-confidence, as well as to improve physical stamina, suppleness, and sense of balance.

YOGA

Yoga, developed in India more than 5,000 years ago, is a system of personal development encompassing body, mind, and spirit. Today many people practice yoga mainly for general health benefits, both preventive and curative. There are many types, but Hatha yoga is the form most well known and commonly practiced in the West. It includes exercises involving special body poses, or *asanas*, controlled breathing techniques, and meditation.

Yogis, or teachers, consider yoga to be but one aspect of attaining enlightenment. According to their teachings, care of the body is less important than spiritual awareness because the body is mortal, whereas the soul is immortal. The ultimate aim of yoga is to unite the human soul with the universal spirit. It is not necessary to accept this philosophy to experience many of yoga's benefits, however. The integrated mind-and-body discipline seems to naturally enhance both physical and mental health and promote mental peace and tranquillity.

Yoga is suitable for people of all ages and fitness levels and offers many therapeutic benefits, including promotion of suppleness, muscular endurance, and relaxation.

Getting started
Yoga develops flexibility and muscular endurance. It can also relieve such mental states as anxiety, depression, and stress, as well as some physical disorders.

Technique is very important; it is advisable to find a qualified teacher—perhaps by personal recommendation. For a yoga class wear loose, comfortable clothing; feet are usually bare. A mat or folded blanket is useful for some exercises.

Yoga tips

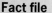

▶ *Never force your limbs or muscles into any position. The flexibility required for more advanced poses will come with practice.*

▶ *Yoga calls for concentrating on breathing and relaxation, as well as the proper forming of the positions.*

Fact file
The word *yoga* comes from the Sanskrit *yug*, meaning "to yoke, or join together." It refers to the union of mind, body, and spirit.

Preparation and safety

Some terms used in yoga describe aspects of its philosophy, and it is useful to know their meanings before you begin. Asanas are body positions in which one aims to remain steady and comfortable, both physically and mentally; the poses help the muscles to become more stretched and flexible and improve the circulation.

Pranayama is the control and direction of vital energy by steady breathing. It increases the energy (prana) in the body, leading to good health.

Meditation is a way of achieving inner peace; thoughts are blocked by focusing the mind on breathing, on an object like a candle, or on a mental image of a favorite place. Some people also play a tape of music or natural sounds or chant a mantra, a constantly repeated phrase or sound.

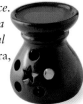

T'AI CHI

T'ai chi chuan, more often referred to as t'ai chi, is both a self-defense strategy and a gentle exercise. In Chinese the words mean "supreme ultimate fist." It was influenced by Taoism, a Chinese philosophy in which all things are considered to be a combination of two forces: *yin*, representing gentle, submissive, feminine qualities, and *yang*, denoting firm, active, masculine aspects. T'ai chi exercises embody the two forces.

T'ai chi is practiced in China and elsewhere in the world today for its numerous health and psychological benefits. Though not as physically demanding as some other martial arts, t'ai chi takes a long time to master. It consists of a series of coordinated exercises, known as a form, based on the movements of certain animals. Forms vary in complexity from 18 postures to more than 100, with all postures flowing together to become one slow, graceful movement. The exercises increase range of movement, correct balance and posture, promote relaxation, and reduce stress. They are coordinated with breathing to encourage *chi*, the body's energy, to flow freely through the energy pathways, or meridians, in the body and aid mental, emotional, and spiritual development.

In China and increasingly in the West, practitioners gather to perform t'ai chi in public parks, often early in the morning, when chi is believed to flow most strongly.

Getting started

T'ai chi cannot be self taught, so the first step is to find a qualified teacher and enroll in a series of classes. It is not necessary to prepare yourself physically before enrolling in t'ai chi classes because the basic exercises are slow and undemanding.

Many people take up t'ai chi to help alleviate a long-standing health problem, such as back pain, and it is

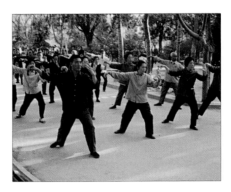

GROUP EXERCISE
Practicing t'ai chi in large groups in parks or other open spaces is a regular morning ritual for many Chinese people.

a good idea to tell the teacher in advance if you have a particular physical condition that needs to be taken into account. The teacher can then help you pace your practice to avoid injury or exacerbation of the problem.

T'ai chi tips

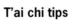

▶ *Correct posture is vital in t'ai chi—the stance should be relaxed, not static or stiff, so that all movements can flow gracefully.*

▶ *Keep your weight evenly balanced over your feet and your knees slightly flexed.*

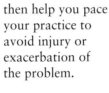

T'ai chi promotes suppleness and muscular strength and is believed to have many therapeutic benefits. It is particularly beneficial for people who have been inactive for a long period.

THE T'AI CHI HAND

T'ai chi focuses on finding a point where balance and harmony are reached. The action of the hands during movements is very important.

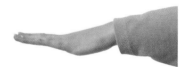

HARSH HAND
If the hands are too stiff and tense, they make movements awkward and limit the flow.

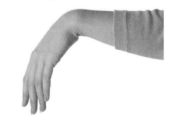

WEAK HAND
If the hands are too lifeless and limp, they drag and detract from the movements.

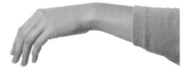

CORRECT POSITION
Ideally in t'ai chi the hands and wrists are relaxed and open, moving easily and gracefully.

Fact file
The roots of t'ai chi are obscure. One account credits its origin to a 13th-century monk who noted that a snake fended off a bird's attack with swift but subtle movements.

JUDO

Judo has its roots in the fighting system of feudal Japan. It developed from the art of ju-jitsu, the original form of hand-to-hand combat practiced by the Samurai, which enabled them to carry on fighting even when deprived of a weapon.

Judo is a wrestling sport that attempts to turn an attacker's force to one's own advantage. Skill, technique, and timing, rather than brute strength, are the essential ingredients for success. Judo teaches flexibility, balance, and the efficient use of leverage and movement in the performance and execution of its throws, grappling techniques, and submission holds.

As a competitive sport, judo offers the opportunity to compete at all skill levels, from club to national tournaments, right up to the Olympic Games, in which it was first included in 1964. The competitors are separated into weight divisions for men, women, boys, and girls. Many people over 60 years of age enjoy the sport, as well as young children and some disabled people.

Getting started

To learn judo, you must find a qualified instructor and join a club or class. You can check in the Yellow Pages and with health clubs to find organizations in the area. During your first lesson you will probably be instructed in some of the history of judo and given an explanation of the modern grading system. You will also do some stretching exercises before you begin. Your instructor will next introduce you to the throwing, grappling, and strangleholds that make up the sport.

Judo helps to boost confidence and enhances a sense of self-reliance, as well as aiding strength and flexibility. To develop all-round fitness, it must be combined with other exercises.

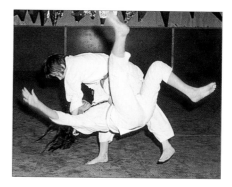

BREAKFALL
One of the first things you will be taught during ukemi *(falling practice) is how to land safely when thrown. It is the most important aspect of judo and reduces the risk of injury during a bout.*

Preparation and safety

When you begin to learn judo, you must expect to rank at the bottom of the group. How well and quickly you progress is up to you. Judo created the system of ranks, now used in most other martial arts, that recognize a person's degree of knowledge, ability, and leadership. There are separate ranks for juniors (under 17 years of age) and seniors. Judo ranks are identified by seven colored belts and a further 10 degrees of advanced status for black belts.

White belt indicates a novice.

Yellow belt represents the end of initial training.

Green and **red** belts show advanced skills.

Blue and **brown** belts denote high accomplishment.

Black belts are worn by masters in the art of judo.

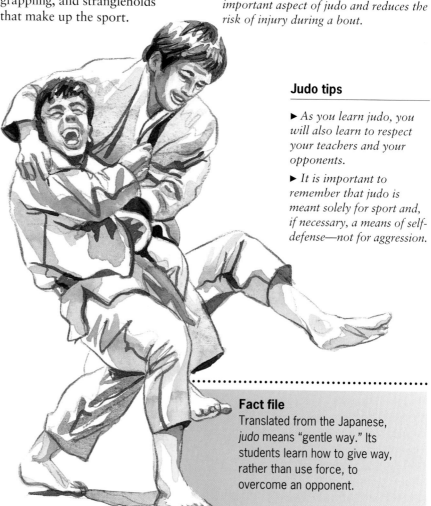

Judo tips

▶ *As you learn judo, you will also learn to respect your teachers and your opponents.*

▶ *It is important to remember that judo is meant solely for sport and, if necessary, a means of self-defense—not for aggression.*

Fact file

Translated from the Japanese, *judo* means "gentle way." Its students learn how to give way, rather than use force, to overcome an opponent.

KARATE

Karate, which means "empty hand" in Japanese, refers broadly to any weaponless Asian martial art, but more specifically to the forms that developed on the island of Okinawa before it became part of the Japanese empire in the late 19th century. The art spread to the Japanese mainland in the early 20th century and from there to many Western countries.

Karate involves executing blows with the feet and hands in coordination with special breathing techniques. Blows can be directed against an opponent or inanimate objects, such as wooden blocks. Taught as a self-defense skill, a competitive sport, and a free-style exercise, karate emphasizes self-discipline, a positive attitude, and high moral purpose. Students of karate are taught to respect both the fighting art and its participants, who may be any age or gender. Karate has a strong Budhist influence; it trains body and mind together. Speed, strength, and technique, along with concentration and focusing of energy, are vital to skillful execution.

Karate students work out barefoot, beginning each class with a few minutes of meditation, then doing some stretching and calisthenics to warm up. Next comes practicing of basic stances, kicks, punches, strikes, and blocks, stopping blows just short of contact. The rest of the time is spent learning *katas*, or forms, which take many years of practice to perfect.

Getting started

As a first step, get a list of all the recognized clubs in your area and find out if their teachers are members of the national governing body for karate. You can be sure then that any grading you are awarded by the club will be accepted by other national bodies.

Decide which style of karate you wish to undertake (see left); some styles may not suit you. Visit different clubs or studios, look at the style, and watch the instructors to observe their teaching methods.

Once you have decided on a club, try it out for a couple of sessions before committing to fees or investing in a karate suit.

KARATE STYLES

The exact evolution of karate is obscure, but it is believed to be based largely on Chinese martial arts blended with early Okinawan techniques. As it spread, karate split into distinct styles, and there is now a wide variety, including a Korean version, tae kwan do. Some styles incorporate elements of Eastern philosophy; others concentrate more on physical aspects. Some are also more aggressive. Kyoku-shinkai, for example, allows punches and kicks to land on the upper body during competition and even permits kicks to the head. This style also puts great store in the ability of exponents to break blocks of wood or stone. Goju, on the other hand, is a more gentle, flowing style in which practitioners counter a hard blow with a soft deflection.

Karate enhances muscular endurance and strength and helps to develop self-discipline. However, training is rigorous and demanding and requires commitment and motivation.

What you will need

The most important piece of equipment will be your suit, or gi. Loose enough to allow free movement yet not baggy or misshapen, the gi has much ritual and history associated with its wearing.

Karate tips

▶ *To gain the most benefit from karate and reduce the risk of injury, regular workouts that develop endurance, strength, and flexibility are necessary.*

▶ *The sudden, rapid, and focused actions of karate depend on holding an easy, relaxed stance, with the knees flexed and the weight of body evenly balanced over the feet.*

Fact file

Karate training includes learning a series of traditional techniques performed in sequence, called katas. There are more than 50 katas to learn, all of which have been preserved from the early masters.

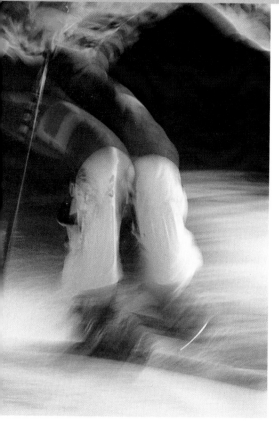

Other Sports

Many sports require the purchase or rental of equipment and a special facility at which to do it, such as a club or open water. Your choice of sport, therefore, may be influenced by cost and the availability of a suitable facility in your area.

BOWLING

Bowling is an ancient game that has been played in some form since at least 5000 B.C. In North America the most popular version is the one played indoors, also called 10-pin bowling (see right). The outdoor game, lawn bowling, has long been steryotyped as a senior's game, but it is attracting more and more young people. Either version will improve strength, balance, and coordination.

Getting started
Both lawn bowling and 10-pin bowling are easy to learn, but they become more rewarding as your skills grow. The balls and special shoes needed for 10-pin bowling can usually be rented wherever the game is played.

Lawn bowling tips

▶ *Hold the bowl with the fingers underneath and avoid gripping it too tightly.*

▶ *Use your body to supply the impetus while your arm mainly guides the direction.*

▶ *Develop an easy, relaxed swing and follow through smoothly with the arm.*

Lawn bowling offers gentle, all-round exercise in the open air and is ideal for less active people. Both lawn and 10-pin bowling are sociable sports that can be enjoyed by the whole family.

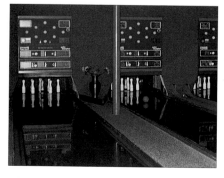

TEN-PIN BOWLING
The indoor sport of 10-pin bowling enjoys widespread popularity. The aim is to knock down 10 pins by rolling a ball along a wooden alley. The game is often played competitively, both individually and in teams.

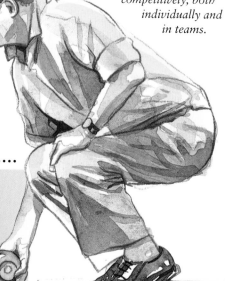

Preparation and safety

Before you begin a game, always have a thorough warm-up and include stretches for the hamstrings, thighs, and lower back because there is a lot of bending and controlled lunging involved.

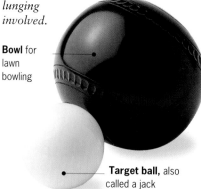

Bowl for lawn bowling

Target ball, also called a jack

USING THE BIAS
A bowl is designed to veer to one side near the end of a run so it can approach the jack from the left or right. Skillful players use this bias to great effect.

Fact file
According to popular legend, in 1588 Sir Francis Drake insisted on finishing his game of bowls before turning his attention to the approaching Spanish Armada. He lost the game but won the battle.

GOLF

The growing popularity of golf may be due to the fact that it combines many different elements. It provides all-round exercise in the open air in pleasant surroundings, and there is a strong element of skill involved. The game affords social opportunities and can be played competitively, but it can also be played alone.

Getting started

Even at a basic level golf requires a fairly high financial commitment. For example, to get the most benefit from golf, you will need lessons with a professional instructor to develop the basic skills—especially the grip and the swing.

You do not have to be a member of a private club to play because there are many municipal courses available. Even so, fees for use of a green and the rental of golf clubs add to the expense. If you decide to join a private club and buy your own set of golf clubs, the sport can become very expensive.

Preparation and safety

Golf can be played with just a few basic clubs. The steeper the angle of the club's head, the farther the ball will travel.

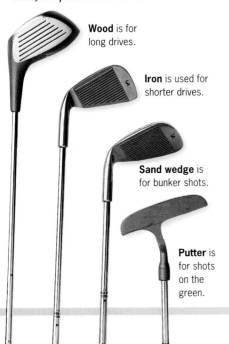

Wood is for long drives.

Iron is used for shorter drives.

Sand wedge is for bunker shots.

Putter is for shots on the green.

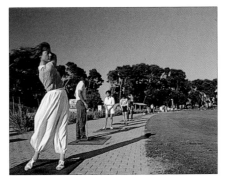

ON THE RANGE
One of the best ways to develop the fitness and skills necessary for golf is to go out and practice on a driving range.

A moderate level of aerobic fitness is needed to delay fatigue and walk the course at a pace that does not obstruct following players. Until such fitness develops, it may be

Golf tips

▶ To *develop a good swing, keep the arms, shoulders, back, and hands relaxed and loose and the legs, knees, and feet flexed and springy.*

▶ *You need flexibility and strength in the shoulders and trunk to create a smooth twisting action in the swing.*

Golf provides all-round fitness benefits but demands commitment in terms of finance, time, training, practice, and motivation in order to develop any amount of skill.

necessary to use a golf cart. To play golf proficiently, a player must develop the power and expertise to drive a ball accurately and repeatedly over varied distances during a game. Power in the upper body, especially the trunk and shoulders, is needed to drive the ball a reasonable distance, and muscular endurance is required to repeat the shot at each hole.

A golfer must also develop isometric (static) strength in order to maintain a correct body position. At the end of a golf swing, the club head is traveling at a great speed, so sufficient strength to slow down the club before damaging the shoulder joint is crucial, especially when a player is becoming tired.

A balanced exercise program, aimed at developing strength and flexibility in the upper body plus aerobic endurance, will help delay fatigue during a day's play and speed recovery after a game.

Walking is an appropriate activity for building aerobic fitness; running, cycling, swimming, and rowing are also useful. Swimming, especially, may aid in the development of flexibility. A general strength training program, using free weights or fixed resistance machines, may aid the golfer initially. A weight-training program that is specific to golf may be more helpful in the longer term.

Fact file
The birthplace of the modern game was St. Andrews, Scotland, which has a course dating from 1754. However, it is thought that the Dutch played a game similar to golf, called *kolf*, around 1300.

ICE SKATING

Ice skating is popular both as a sport and as a recreational pastime. Each individual can make time on the ice as challenging as he or she wishes by enjoying gentle exercise, practicing speed skating, or learning the more advanced jumps and dance movements used for figure skating.

Getting started

The number of indoor rinks is growing steadily, and most of them employ coaches who can help with the first steps in learning to skate. Also, some communities in areas where the winters are cold enough monitor and supervise skating on a local pond or lake.

The techniques necessary for ice skating are good for developing strength in the leg and gluteal muscles. The sport also develops a keen sense of balance and improves posture. Cycling, running, or rowing

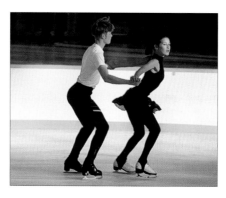

SKATING LESSONS
You can often find professional coaches who are affiliated with a particular ice rink and offer instruction to individuals or small groups.

combined with resistance training are excellent methods of preparing for skating because they strengthen the muscles and increase stamina, which is required for all forms of skating. Sprinting practice is helpful for ice dance and figure skating,

Ice skating is an enjoyable and sociable sport that requires little financial outlay. It provides good cardiovascular exercise and is ideal for strengthening the leg muscles.

while endurance training is more useful for speed skating. Ice dancing and figure skating also benefit from dance training, which enhances suppleness and ease of movement. The only special equipment required is well-fitting skates. Most rinks rent skates, so you can decide if you like the sport before investing in your own pair. You don't have to accept the first pair of skates the rink offers you. If they are at all uncomfortable or otherwise unacceptable, exchange them. Ice skates should fit very snugly, permitting the foot very little room to move within the boot.

Skating at an ice rink

There are certain rules to follow when rink skating. Always skate counterclockwise around the edge of the rink—the center area is usually reserved for people practicing figure skating maneuvers—and be aware of other skaters. It is advisable to wear gloves at all times and for children under five years to wear some form of head protection, such as an ice

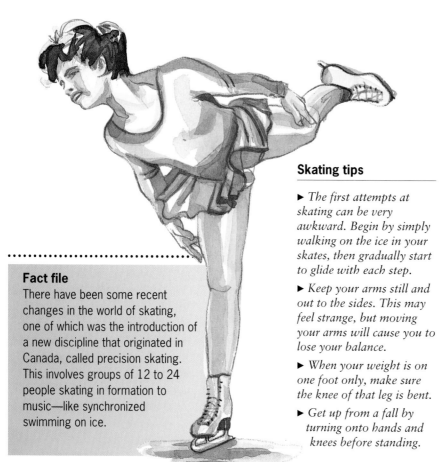

Fact file
There have been some recent changes in the world of skating, one of which was the introduction of a new discipline that originated in Canada, called precision skating. This involves groups of 12 to 24 people skating in formation to music—like synchronized swimming on ice.

Skating tips

▶ *The first attempts at skating can be very awkward. Begin by simply walking on the ice in your skates, then gradually start to glide with each step.*

▶ *Keep your arms still and out to the sides. This may feel strange, but moving your arms will cause you to lose your balance.*

▶ *When your weight is on one foot only, make sure the knee of that leg is bent.*

▶ *Get up from a fall by turning onto hands and knees before standing.*

Preparation and safety

The essential piece of equipment is a snug-fitting pair of ice skates. The skates should support your ankle and instep and should neither slip around on your foot nor pinch it. The blades should be clean and the edges sharp. Bear in mind that an ice skate blade can be very sharp, so protect your fingers when learning to skate and wear thick warm clothing. A beginner tends to spend quite some time sitting on the ice! To test your blades for sharpness, run your fingernail along each edge. If the blades scrape a little of your nail away, they have an edge; if not, they need sharpening.

hockey helmet. You should not wear such loose articles of clothing as scarves or carry other droppable items like drinks or personal stereos onto the ice. Anything you drop may become a hazard to other skaters.

Skating on open ice

Skating on natural ice, such as a frozen lake or pond, can be dangerous unless it has been certified safe for skating; the ice may not be consistently solid enough to support your weight and could give way without warning. Never skate on ice if you can't be certain of its thickness; even when you are sure ice is safe, it's best to skate with a partner.

ICE HOCKEY

Ice hockey is a highly skilled and popular game that combines the strength and balance of the skater with the hand-eye coordination of the hockey player. The techniques and training necessary for ice skating require powerful lower body muscles plus good upper body strength for stick work. The initial financial outlay is high because of the cost of special ice hockey boots, the stick, and protective gear.

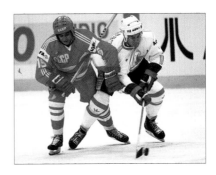

ICE HOCKEY
The protective clothing worn by ice hockey players gives an indication of the physical nature of the sport.

ROLLER SKATING

Roller skating is an adaptation of ice skating that has become popular worldwide. It is a year-round, accessible, and fun way to exercise that can be enjoyed by the whole family. Most people take up roller skating informally as children and then grow out of the sport, but many young adults are returning to it.

Roller skating can be done virtually anywhere that is away from traffic and does not put pedestrians at risk. The sport is excellent for developing balance, stamina, and strength in the leg and gluteal

muscles. Dancing, cycling, and weight training can help build up the fitness and strength you will need to get the most out of roller skating.

Roller Blades, or in-line skates, the latest innovation in roller skating, were invented as a summer training device for ice hockey players. They are more difficult to master because the wheels are in a line like the blades of ice skates rather than positioned at the four corners. It's possible to attain greater speed and maneuverability with these skates, but they are also more difficult to master.

Getting started

The skills necessary to take the first steps are fairly easy to acquire, and with practice, skating ability and confidence increase quickly. Just as in ice skating, there is scope for serious devotees to get involved in competitive events. The four main types of roller-skating competition are artistic skating, speed skating, roller-skate hockey, and roller derby—a speed-skating event staged on a banked track.

Although roller skates should not be as tight fitting as ice skates, they should be snug. It is strongly recommended that you wear

Apart from the purchase of roller skates and a modicum of protective gear, there is little expense involved, and the sport offers good all-round cardiovascular and strength exercise.

protective padding on your knees and elbows when roller skating and also wear a protective helmet—especially if you are skating on concrete or other hard surfaces. Every year many people sustain serious injuries in skating accidents, particularly with in-line skates.

Preparation and safety

In-line skates should support your ankle and instep, just like ice skates, and should neither slip nor pinch.

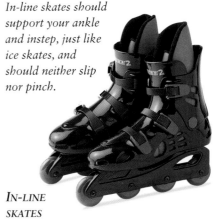

IN-LINE SKATES
The wheels should be cleaned periodically to keep them free of anything that might affect their movement.

ROLLER BLADING
The popularity of roller blading as a sport in its own right has grown immensely in recent years, and the skills and fancy maneuvers of its devotees are growing ever more incredible.

SKIING

Skiing is an exhilarating but physically demanding sport; it requires a high level of aerobic fitness and plenty of strength in the upper body and the legs. Skiing is also very expensive, so to make the most of your time on the slopes, it is sensible to prepare yourself in advance.

Getting started

Before going on a skiing holiday—or even taking skiing lessons at a dry ski slope—it is advisable to work on strength, endurance, and flexibility. The best physical preparation for skiing is to use an indoor ski simulator machine, which is designed to strengthen all the muscles you use

when skiing. Alternatively, you can plan your own tailor-made workout to achieve a similar effect. The crouched stance that is used in skiing can be very demanding on the thigh muscles, so your workout should focus particular attention on this area of the body. Step training, cycling, or jogging will improve your strength and endurance, particularly in the large muscles of the legs.

As a beginner, you will also need to develop your upper body strength. First-time skiers tend to fall over a lot, so they are constantly having to push themselves back up to a standing position.

Skiing on vacation

Skiing is the most popular winter holiday activity, but people often set off without adequate preparation. There are many aspects of skiing that can prove far more demanding than you might expect. Being unprepared means you will quickly become exhausted and increase your risk of injury. Most ski resorts have instructors for all levels of ability; signing up for lessons will ensure that you learn the basics sufficiently to enjoy the sport in reasonable safety, but you shouldn't take unnecessary risks. In particular, avoid ski slopes that are beyond your level of skiing ability.

Skiing, an invigorating and highly sociable sport, is expensive. However, it offers a good incentive to get fit beforehand and can be enjoyed by people of any age.

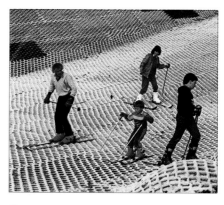

DRY SKI SLOPES
Practicing on dry ski slopes before you venture onto snow-covered ones can help you master the basics without having to devote the first part of your holiday to learning how to stand and fall safely.

Skiing tips

▶ *Keep your feet hip width apart and press your weight down on the whole length of both feet to help you stay balanced.*

▶ *Keep your knees slightly bent and steer with your feet, not with your shoulders.*

Preparation and safety

Ski equipment is expensive, so most people rent their equipment at first. Make sure the ski boots you use fit well and provide good ankle support while still allowing normal bending and straightening. At mountain altitudes, more ultraviolet rays from the sun reach you than at sea level, so always use a sun block with an SPF factor of at least 15, higher if you are sensitive to sunlight.

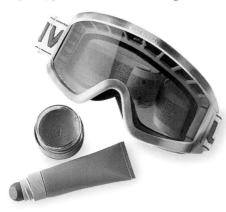

SUN PROTECTION
In addition to protecting yourself from the cold, you must also shield your eyes and skin from the sun. Wear protective goggles and apply sun block to exposed skin. A mixture of sun and wind may chap your lips, so lip salve is also recommended.

Fact file

The word *ski* comes from the Norwegian for snowshoe. The earliest references to skiing date back to 2500 B.C.

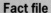

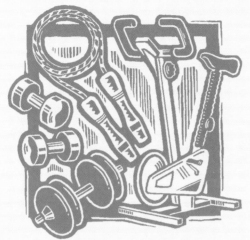

CHAPTER 7

EXERCISE AT HOME AND IN THE OFFICE

A problem that many people face when trying to increase their exercise is how to incorporate regular sessions into a life that is already too busy. With a little planning and small changes in habits, you can turn your home and even your office into highly effective fitness centers.

SETTING UP A HOME GYM

Although budget and available space are major considerations when setting up a home gym, the most important thing to consider is exactly what it is you want and need from it.

If you want to see positive results from a physical exercise program, it is essential to keep it going. The convenience of having your own gym at home may help you stay with your fitness regimen. Setting up your own home gym can also be great fun and ultimately very rewarding.

Once the initial investment has been made, there are no further costs, whereas attending a health club requires annual or monthly membership fees and travel expenses. A home gym needn't break the bank, however; it is possible to utilize many household items (see opposite page).

Lack of time is often used as an excuse not to exercise. With a home gym no time is wasted traveling, and its use is not restricted to certain hours of the day. Exercising at home has the added advantage of privacy, and you can listen to your own choice of music. A home gym also offers an ideal way to encourage the whole family to do more exercise. Creating the opportunity to exercise together will not only improve health and fitness but also help strengthen family bonds.

Older members of the family may benefit particularly from exercise equipment that is designed to improve aerobic, or cardiovascular, fitness. You should make sure, however, to set it at the least strenuous level when using it for the first time and to increase the difficulty very gradually, only when fitness levels have clearly improved. Strength-training equipment can be unsuitable for people who have high blood pressure. They should use it only after seeking the advice of their doctor.

Children should not attempt to use weights before their early teens because their bones are soft and easily damaged. Most exercise machines are also unsuitable for young children, but they can enjoy using simple pieces of gym equipment, such as a jump rope or trampoline. Aim to keep the exercise sessions short because a small child's attention span is limited. The focus should be on physical play so that exercise is fun for the child. Examples are playing tag in the garden or including simple aerobic actions in a game like Simon Says, which the child can try to mimic. Stretching and floor exercises are also very good for youngsters, especially when done to music.

Older children can be encouraged to use more sophisticated pieces of gym equipment if you have them, but you must make sure they know how to use them properly and are supervised at all times.

FACTORS TO CONSIDER
A home gym does not have to involve the purchase of complicated and expensive equipment. For some people clearing a space on the living room floor and exercising to an aerobic workout video will be enough to increase their levels of fitness.

FAMILY FITNESS
Holding regular exercise sessions in your own home will encourage the whole family to get into the fitness habit.

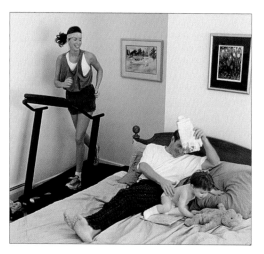

An Inexpensive Home Gym

You don't have to spend a fortune on exercise machines in order to keep fit in the comfort of your own home. Some simple items that can be bought quite cheaply make excellent fitness aids, and there are everyday household objects that can also be used as pieces of home exercise equipment.

Cans of food

Various sizes of food cans can double as dumbbells for exercises such as curls, lateral raises, and dumbbell presses.

Do...develop a smooth, rhythmical movement.

Do...stand straight with your feet shoulder width apart.

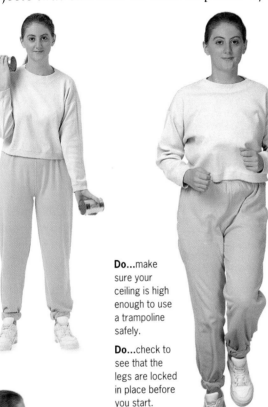

Skipping rope

Skipping provides excellent aerobic exercise. You can buy a jump rope or use a length of rope from the hardware store. Start with sets of 20 to 30 skips at a time and rest for a minute between sets. As you progress, build up to 60 to 100 skips a minute for up to 20 minutes.

Do...wear cushioned trainers.

Don't...skip on hard surfaces.

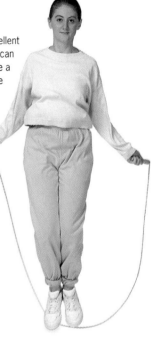

Do...make sure your ceiling is high enough to use a trampoline safely.

Do...check to see that the legs are locked in place before you start.

Do...use a sturdy table.

Do...keep your back straight.

Don't...lock your knees.

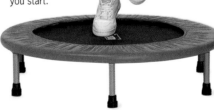

Baby trampoline

A trampoline can enhance aerobic fitness and also provide low-impact, weight-bearing exercise to strengthen muscles and bones.

Stairs

Using your own stairs regularly provides good aerobic and weight-bearing exercise. You can use the bottom stair for aerobic step routines. Alternatively, use a sturdy wooden box or bench.

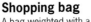
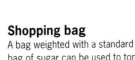

Shopping bag

A bag weighted with a standard bag of sugar can be used to tone and strengthen the leg muscles.

Stairs

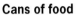

HERBED CHEESE & ONION POTATO BREAD

This delicious cheese, onion, and potato-filled loaf is full of complex carbohydrates for energy. Enjoy a piece before your next exercise session to keep you fueled.

425 ml (1¾ cups) vegetable stock, lukewarm
25 g (1 oz) Parmesan cheese, grated (¼ cup)
2 tbsp olive oil
2 tbsp honey
1 tbsp chopped parsley
1 tbsp chopped chives
2 tbsp active dry yeast
300 g (11 oz) mashed potato (about 1¼ cups)
400 g (3 cups) bread flour or all-purpose flour
400 g (3 cups) whole-wheat flour
½ tsp salt
½ small onion, grated

- In a large bowl, mix the stock, Parmesan, oil, honey, parsley, and chives, then gently stir in the yeast. Stir in the mashed potato. Set aside for 10 minutes or until the mixture foams.
- In another large bowl, mix the flours and salt. Gradually stir 550 g (4 cups) of the flours and the grated onion into the potato mixture.
- Turn the dough onto a floured surface; knead in the remaining flour. Continue kneading for 10 minutes or until elastic in consistency.
- Lightly grease the bowl with olive oil. Add the dough, coating it with oil on all sides. Cover the bowl with a damp towel and allow dough to rise in a warm, draft-free place for 30 to 40 minutes or until doubled in size.
- Punch the dough back down into the bowl and knead for 1 minute. Divide the dough in half and shape into two loaves.
- Lightly grease two 21 × 11 cm (8½ × 4½ in) loaf pans. Add the dough, cover, and allow loaves to rise in a warm place for 30 minutes or until doubled in size.
- Preheat the oven to 180°C/350°F. Bake for 30 minutes or until the loaves sound hollow when tapped. Cool on wire racks for 30 minutes.

Makes 2 loaves

However, you may feel the need for a more sophisticated setup, either because you want a more comprehensive workout or because you would like to alleviate the monotony of doing the same exercises over and over. Before you start purchasing equipment to use at home, however, it is important to consider what it is you want to achieve, how much you can afford to spend, and the amount of space you have available.

Deciding on your fitness objectives

You have to decide whether you want just to get aerobically fit, build up your strength, or increase your flexibility, or if you want to achieve a mixture of all three. These factors will determine what kind of equipment you have to buy. For example, if you want a machine that will give you a cardiovascular workout but do not want to do any resistance training, a simple exercise bike or treadmill will meet your needs. If, however, you want to build your strength as well as get aerobically fit, you will also need a set of weights or some resistance machinery.

Whatever your objectives, the most basic requirement of any home gym is a good-quality exercise mat on which to stretch and do floor exercises. A mat cushions and reduces the impact on your joints and makes floor work much more comfortable.

Cost

Figure out how much money you have to spend; there is no point in planning a huge multigym if you have a limited budget. Remember that your gym can start small and grow as your finances do. Obviously, the more money you have, the more comprehensive your gym can be, but you can pick up the necessary equipment less expensively to begin with by seeking the advice of professionals and shopping around.

It is important to know what type of equipment you are going to need to meet your exercise goals. Buying inappropriate equipment is costly and frustrating. To make the correct choice, start by reading about what is available. If possible, test various pieces of equipment and machinery at your local health club to see what suits you and will keep you motivated to exercise in the long term. Go into a sports store and speak to trained sales assistants about your needs and keep a lookout for any special offers. Remember, if you don't like a piece of equipment at your health club, you won't like it in your own home.

Available space

Think about the space you have available. The inconvenience of having to set up each time and move heavy furniture may tempt you to skip sessions. Make sure you have ample room in which to exercise and that your space is well ventilated and free of electrical wires or appliances that might lead to injury while you are exercising.

A full-length mirror can be useful for monitoring technique and for motivation. Also, when planning your gym, take into account the height of your ceilings; some pieces of equipment, such as multigyms, can be quite tall. If the equipment is heavy, make sure that the floor or supporting walls are strong enough to accommodate the weight.

Finally, consider whether you have room enough to expand your gym as you become more proficient with the machinery you have and perhaps want to purchase additional equipment. You might keep various pieces of gym equipment in different rooms or in a cellar, garage, or shed. Make sure any room you use can be kept warm and draft-free because a cold environment is likely to discourage you from exercising and will increase the risk of injuries, such as strains and sprains.

STRENGTH-TRAINING MACHINERY

If you desire to increase your strength, power, and endurance or build up your muscles, you will benefit from such devices as an exercise bench, free weights, like barbells and dumbbells, and/or fixed-weight machinery, such as a multigym.

Exercise bench

An exercise bench is an invaluable addition to a home exercise setup, particularly if it is adjustable. It is useful not only for weight training but also for supporting abdominal exercises, tricep dips, and push-ups.

Free weights

A basic set of free weights, including a barbell and a pair of dumbbells, is all you need for a resistance workout (see page 130).

A barbell is a hollow or solid steel bar about 1 to 2 meters (3 to 6 feet) in length. Pairs of weights, known as plates, which weigh from as little as you choose to as heavy as you can safely manage to lift, are attached to the ends of the bar and held in place with collars.

Dumbbells are like short barbells, 25 to 40 centimeters (10 to 16 inches) long. Some are one piece and come in sets of varying weights; others are adjustable, like barbells,

CORRECT WEIGHT-LIFTING TECHNIQUE

The most important aspect of resistance training with a barbell is to use the correct lifting technique at all times. This involves adopting the proper body posture, the correct foot positioning, and a suitable grip. When you have successfully lifted the weight, you should carry out all exercises with it using a smooth, even rhythm. Always breathe out on the most physically exerting phase of the exercise. Concentrate on breathing evenly to keep your blood pressure steady. Reverse the sequence shown when returning the bar to the floor.

USING BARBELLS SAFELY

Grip the bar with your thumb under the weight and your knuckles above. Hold the bar to either side of your feet, keeping your wrists straight and locked to avoid strain or injury.

Keep your back in a straight line at all times and bend only your knees; this way your leg muscles bear most of the weight.

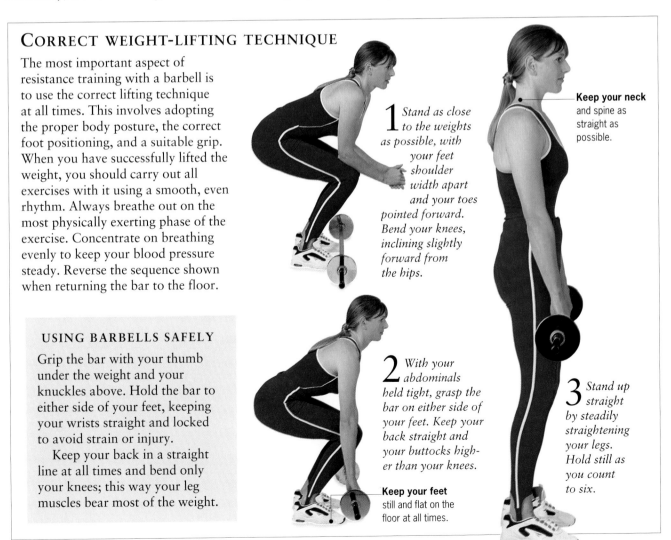

1 *Stand as close to the weights as possible, with your feet shoulder width apart and your toes pointed forward. Bend your knees, inclining slightly forward from the hips.*

2 *With your abdominals held tight, grasp the bar on either side of your feet. Keep your back straight and your buttocks higher than your knees.*

Keep your feet still and flat on the floor at all times.

Keep your neck and spine as straight as possible.

3 *Stand up straight by steadily straightening your legs. Hold still as you count to six.*

123

WEIGHT SAFETY

Before you begin each weight-training session, follow these few tips for a safer workout.

▶ *Make sure children and pets are out of the room while you train. Always keep weights out of the reach of children.*

▶ *Remove fragile objects from your training area.*

▶ *Don't exercise on days when you are sore or don't feel well.*

▶ *Make sure that all collars or clips holding the weight plates in place are secure before lifting.*

▶ *Begin every training session with a thorough warm-up and finish with a cool-down and stretches (see page 70).*

CAUTION

People who suffer from high blood pressure or from back or joint problems should always consult a doctor before doing any weight-lifting exercises. If your doctor deems them unsuitable, there are still many other toning exercises that you can do to stay fit and increase your strength.

so that you can add plates to them to increase the weight. Start with weights that enable you to do the repetitions easily.

Free weights offer the best way for you to isolate individual muscles or muscle groups and work them in a controlled manner to increase muscle growth and strength. Also, if you use lighter weights but do more frequent repetitions, you can improve both suppleness and muscle tone.

The disadvantage of free weights is that you need some degree of training to learn how to control their movement safely and to make the target muscle perform the dominant share of the work. Without good control, the weight cannot be moved along the

correct and safe path, and this can result in injury if excessive stress is placed on a joint or muscle too weak to handle it.

Always seek expert advice before using free weights for the first time, to reduce the risk of accidental injuries and to avoid developing poor exercising techniques that can lead to long-term physical damage.

Fixed-weight machinery

Machines with fixed weights, such as multigyms, perform the same job as free weights but allow you to lift heavier weights without the aid of a training partner and without having to change the plates for each exercise. They also combine lots of different exercises into a single piece of machinery that is safe and easy to use.

A good multigym will allow you to work all the major muscle groups through a system of pulleys attached to a central weight stack. By connecting various attachments and positioning the body in different ways, you can effectively strengthen the muscles of the legs, arms, and torso. When choosing a multigym, shop for one that feels solid and fits your available space. Don't forget to consider the height of your ceiling and the strength of your floor.

BENEFITS OF DUMBBELLS

Dumbbells make ideal home fitness devices because of their great versatility, convenience, and relatively low cost.

Their greatest asset is that they can easily accommodate each individual's physical strength and range of movement. However, they require some initial training for their safe and effective use.

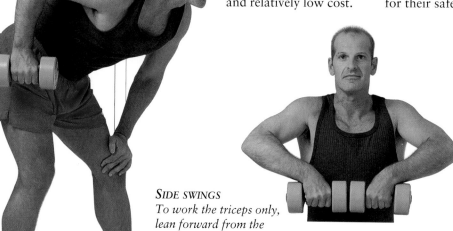

SIDE SWINGS
To work the triceps only, lean forward from the waist, hold a weight by your side, and swing the lower arm forward and backward.

FRONT RAISES
Slowly raise both weights to chest height to work the shoulder muscles.

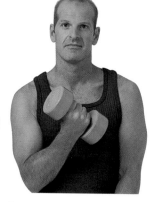

CURLS
To strengthen your biceps and forearms, slowly raise one weight to your shoulder.

YOUR OWN HOME WORKOUT

If you do not have the time or inclination to attend exercise classes, you can plan your own fitness program and have a complete workout at home.

The routines on the following pages are designed to be carried out in the home with just a few pieces of inexpensive equipment. Before you begin a home workout, look carefully at the room in which you've chosen to exercise, making sure that it is safe and free of obstructions. Remove any loose rugs and arrange the furniture for maximum space. Make sure there are no electric or telephone cords in the exercise area. Also check that you have plenty of room above and around you to move your arms; low-hanging ceiling fixtures can be a particular problem.

If your floor is made of concrete overlaid with a single layer of carpet, it is advisable to do any high-impact exercises, such as jogging, in place on your exercise mat.

To balance your weekly exercise regimen and give the different muscle groups time to rest, do cardiovascular exercises and toning exercises on alternate days. Every exercise session must include a warm-up before and a cool-down period afterward. For most people short, regular workouts are easier to maintain than lengthier but less frequent sessions. A full-length mirror can be very useful for checking your technique.

YOUR HOME CIRCUIT

Doing a variety of exercises in a certain sequence, known as circuit training, provides a varied workout for the major muscle groups and the cardiovascular system. A circuit is a series of stations at which different exercises are performed in succession. Each station may focus on cardiovascular and/or resistance exercises, sometimes using various pieces of equipment. It is easy to set up your own circuit at home; just make sure there is nothing to get in your way, such as furniture or trailing electric wires. Plan everything beforehand and be sure to warm up and stretch out properly before you begin (see page 70).

Station 1 ▶ *Stairs: Walk briskly up and down your stairs six times. If you don't have access to stairs, consider buying or making an aerobic step or perform knee lifts (see page 128).*

Station 2 ▶ *Push-ups: Find a clear space on your floor and perform 20 push-ups (see page 131).*

Station 3 ▶ *Curl-ups: Lie on an exercise mat or thick towel and do 20 curl-ups, taking care not to clasp hands tightly behind your head (see page 75).*

Station 4 ▶ *Lunges: Do 10 dumbbell lunges with each leg (see page 130). If you do not have dumbbells, use household objects, such as filled plastic water bottles or cans of soup.*

Station 5 ▶ *Running: Run up and down your garden, around the block, or in place for 2 minutes.*

Station 6 ▶ *Sways: Find a clear space and do 16 sways (see page 128). Alternatively, do 16 half stars (see page 129).*

Station 7 ▶ *Jumping rope: Jump rope for 1 minute. Make sure you have ample room all around and above your head so that the rope can move freely.*

Station 8 ▶ *Chair squats: Squat down onto the edge of a chair slowly, feeling the contraction in your thighs, and then stand up again. Repeat this 20 times.*

▶ *Repeat the circuit at least once more, but for a thorough workout, aim to repeat it as many times as you can for up to 30 minutes.*

Stretching Exercises

You should always stretch before and after any type of exercise, but daily stretching is also beneficial for its own sake because it helps to maintain your full range of movement, reduce tension, improve posture, and prevent injuries.

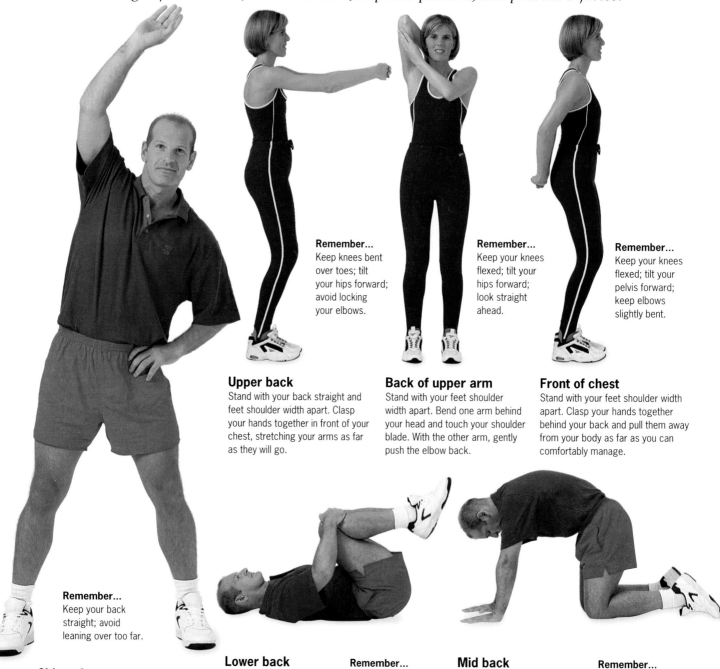

Remember...
Keep knees bent over toes; tilt your hips forward; avoid locking your elbows.

Remember...
Keep your knees flexed; tilt your hips forward; look straight ahead.

Remember...
Keep your knees flexed; tilt your pelvis forward; keep elbows slightly bent.

Upper back
Stand with your back straight and feet shoulder width apart. Clasp your hands together in front of your chest, stretching your arms as far as they will go.

Back of upper arm
Stand with your feet shoulder width apart. Bend one arm behind your head and touch your shoulder blade. With the other arm, gently push the elbow back.

Front of chest
Stand with your feet shoulder width apart. Clasp your hands together behind your back and pull them away from your body as far as you can comfortably manage.

Remember...
Keep your back straight; avoid leaning over too far.

Sides of torso
Stand with your feet well apart and knees slightly bent. Rest one hand on your hip and stretch the other arm up. Lean your torso over to the other side until you feel a slight tension.

Lower back
Lie on your back and raise your knees. Place your hands on your knees and slowly pull them toward your abdomen until you feel the stretch. Hold for 2 seconds.

Remember...
Pull in your stomach muscles tightly; make sure you lower your legs slowly; keep your upper back and shoulders on the mat.

Mid back
Start on all fours, with hands under shoulders and arms slightly bent. Breathe in as you slowly arch your back. Hold for 2 seconds. Breathe out as you reverse movement.

Remember...
Hold your abdominal muscles in and tilt your pelvis forward; avoid locking the elbows; don't over-arch your back.

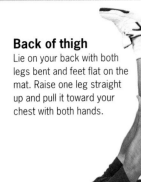

Back of thigh

Lie on your back with both legs bent and feet flat on the mat. Raise one leg straight up and pull it toward your chest with both hands.

Remember...

Keep your lower back on the mat. If you cannot reach the leg, loop a towel around your calf and pull it toward you.

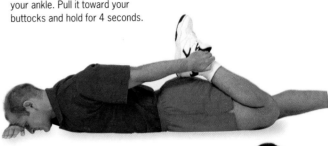

Front of thigh

Lie face down on the mat with your forehead resting on a forearm. Bend one leg behind you and grasp your ankle. Pull it toward your buttocks and hold for 4 seconds.

Remember...

Keep your hips on the mat and your knees together; hold your abdominal muscles in.

Hip flexor

Kneel on the mat and raise your left leg until you can place your foot flat on the mat. Move the right leg back as far as it will comfortably go. Place your hands on your left leg for support. Hold the stretch when you feel mild tension in the upper calf.

Remember...

Keep your head, neck, and spine in line; avoid twisting the knee.

Upper calf

Standing with back straight, stretch one leg back, keeping the other leg slightly bent. Push against the mat with the ball of the back foot until you feel the stretch in the groin.

Remember...

Hold your abdominal muscles in; keep your knees flexed and feet facing forward; push your hips forward.

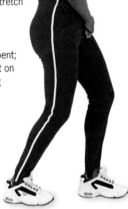

Lower calf

Stand with feet facing forward and move one leg back slightly, keeping both knees bent. Push against the back foot until you feel the stretch in your lower calf.

Remember...

Keep both knees bent; place both feet flat on the mat and facing forward.

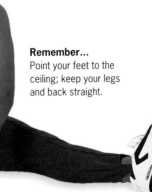

Inner thigh

Sit on the mat with your legs as wide apart as you find comfortable and your hands flat on the mat. Keeping your back straight and abdominal muscles pulled in, reach forward until you feel a slight tension in the inner thighs.

Remember...

Point your feet to the ceiling; keep your legs and back straight.

BE SAFE AND EFFECTIVE

When you are stretching, make sure of the following:

▶ *Muscles must be warm. Before stretching, march in place for a couple of minutes or until your body has warmed up.*

▶ *Move into the stretches slowly and gently and avoid bouncing.*

▶ *Hold stretches for a minimum of 8 to 10 seconds, except when shorter times are given.*

▶ *Stretch to a point of slight tension but not pain.*

▶ *Always do the stretches on both sides of the body for equal lengths of time.*

Aerobic Routine

This routine improves your cardiovascular fitness. For the first few times, aim to exercise for 10 minutes at an intensity that makes you breathe harder than usual yet still allows you to talk. If it feels too hard, slow down and stop.

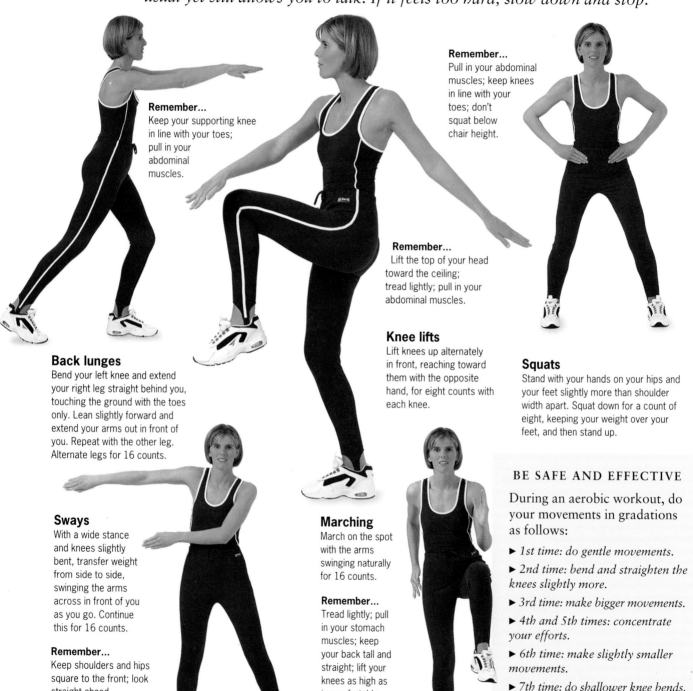

Remember...
Keep your supporting knee in line with your toes; pull in your abdominal muscles.

Remember...
Pull in your abdominal muscles; keep knees in line with your toes; don't squat below chair height.

Remember...
Lift the top of your head toward the ceiling; tread lightly; pull in your abdominal muscles.

Knee lifts
Lift knees up alternately in front, reaching toward them with the opposite hand, for eight counts with each knee.

Back lunges
Bend your left knee and extend your right leg straight behind you, touching the ground with the toes only. Lean slightly forward and extend your arms out in front of you. Repeat with the other leg. Alternate legs for 16 counts.

Squats
Stand with your hands on your hips and your feet slightly more than shoulder width apart. Squat down for a count of eight, keeping your weight over your feet, and then stand up.

Sways
With a wide stance and knees slightly bent, transfer weight from side to side, swinging the arms across in front of you as you go. Continue this for 16 counts.

Remember...
Keep shoulders and hips square to the front; look straight ahead.

Marching
March on the spot with the arms swinging naturally for 16 counts.

Remember...
Tread lightly; pull in your stomach muscles; keep your back tall and straight; lift your knees as high as is comfortable.

BE SAFE AND EFFECTIVE

During an aerobic workout, do your movements in gradations as follows:

▶ *1st time: do gentle movements.*

▶ *2nd time: bend and straighten the knees slightly more.*

▶ *3rd time: make bigger movements.*

▶ *4th and 5th times: concentrate your efforts.*

▶ *6th time: make slightly smaller movements.*

▶ *7th time: do shallower knee bends.*

▶ *8th time: slow down movements and do them gently.*

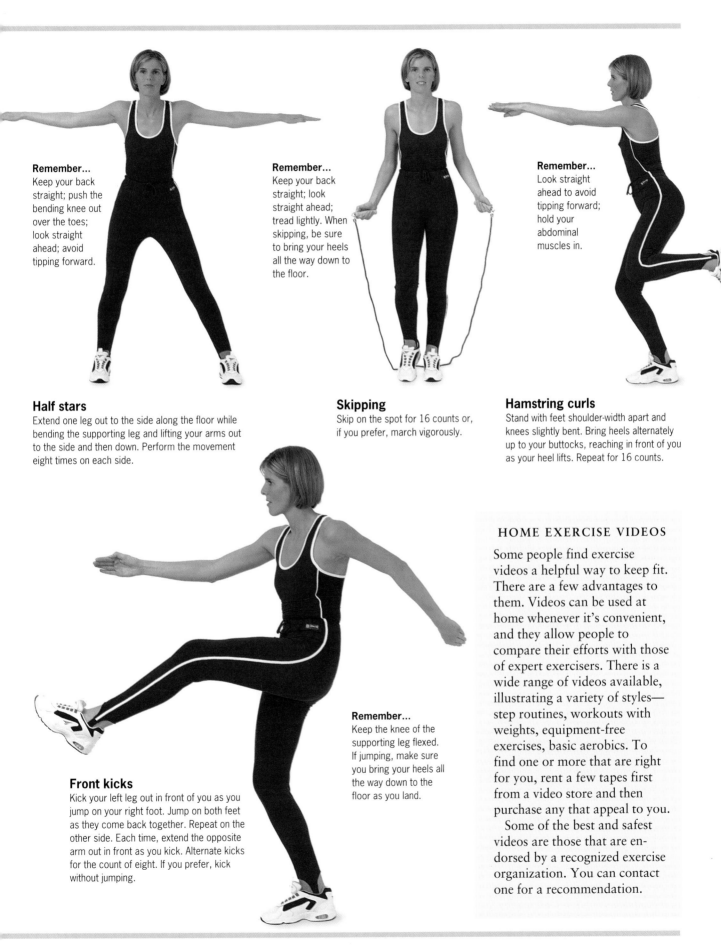

Remember...
Keep your back straight; push the bending knee out over the toes; look straight ahead; avoid tipping forward.

Remember...
Keep your back straight; look straight ahead; tread lightly. When skipping, be sure to bring your heels all the way down to the floor.

Remember...
Look straight ahead to avoid tipping forward; hold your abdominal muscles in.

Half stars
Extend one leg out to the side along the floor while bending the supporting leg and lifting your arms out to the side and then down. Perform the movement eight times on each side.

Skipping
Skip on the spot for 16 counts or, if you prefer, march vigorously.

Hamstring curls
Stand with feet shoulder-width apart and knees slightly bent. Bring heels alternately up to your buttocks, reaching in front of you as your heel lifts. Repeat for 16 counts.

Remember...
Keep the knee of the supporting leg flexed. If jumping, make sure you bring your heels all the way down to the floor as you land.

Front kicks
Kick your left leg out in front of you as you jump on your right foot. Jump on both feet as they come back together. Repeat on the other side. Each time, extend the opposite arm out in front as you kick. Alternate kicks for the count of eight. If you prefer, kick without jumping.

HOME EXERCISE VIDEOS
Some people find exercise videos a helpful way to keep fit. There are a few advantages to them. Videos can be used at home whenever it's convenient, and they allow people to compare their efforts with those of expert exercisers. There is a wide range of videos available, illustrating a variety of styles— step routines, workouts with weights, equipment-free exercises, basic aerobics. To find one or more that are right for you, rent a few tapes first from a video store and then purchase any that appeal to you.

Some of the best and safest videos are those that are endorsed by a recognized exercise organization. You can contact one for a recommendation.

Toning Routine

The following routine will improve your muscular strength and endurance while firming and toning your muscles. You will need weights, such as a set of dumbbells or filled plastic water bottles, and an exercise mat. Initially, aim to complete two sets of 10 repetitions, progressing to three sets of 15.

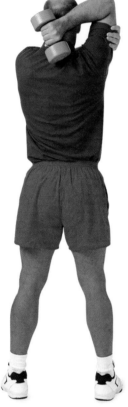

Triceps extension

Works Muscles at the back of the upper arm (triceps)

Stand with your back straight and legs shoulder width apart. Hold a dumbbell in your right hand above your head. Slowly lower the dumbbell behind and across the back of your neck, bending your arm at the elbow. Lift it above your head again but do not return it to the perpendicular (this will force the triceps to work harder).

Remember...
Pull your stomach in and keep your wrist straight but avoid locking the elbow when the arm is straight; alternate arms to work in sets; keep your movements smooth and flowing; keep your weight balanced over your feet.

Torso lift

Works Lower back muscles (erector spinae)

Lie face down with your hands by the side of your head, legs straight, feet together, and toes resting on the mat. Pull your abdominal muscles in, breathe in, and slowly raise your torso off the mat, breathing out as you do so. Hold for 2 seconds and then slowly lower again.

Remember...
Keep your head, neck, and spine in line and your chin down; keep your hips pressed into the mat.

Dumbbell lunge

Works Thighs (quadriceps and hamstrings) and buttocks (gluteals).

Stand with your feet shoulder width apart and weights by your sides. Step forward with the right leg, bending both knees and letting the back heel lift off the floor. Push with the right leg to get back to the starting position. Repeat, this time leading with the left leg.

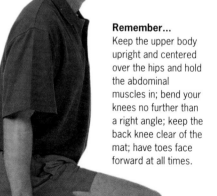

Remember...
Keep the upper body upright and centered over the hips and hold the abdominal muscles in; bend your knees no further than a right angle; keep the back knee clear of the mat; have toes face forward at all times.

Abdominal curl with resistance

Works Abdominal muscles

Lie on your back with knees bent and feet flat on the floor. Hold a weight on your chest. Pull in your abdominal muscles and lift your head and shoulders off the floor as you breathe out. Lower back down to the starting position.

Remember...
Exhale as you curl up; keep your chin in a relaxed and neutral position and your lower back on the mat.

Three-quarter push-up

Works Muscles of the chest (pectorals), upper arms (triceps), and shoulders (anterior deltoids)

Lie face down and place your hands below your shoulders with the palms flat on the floor. Lift your feet off the floor. Breathing out, push your chest off the floor. Hold for a count of two and then breathe in as you lower your body back to the floor.

Remember...
Keep your abdominals pulled in and your back straight; avoid locking your elbows.

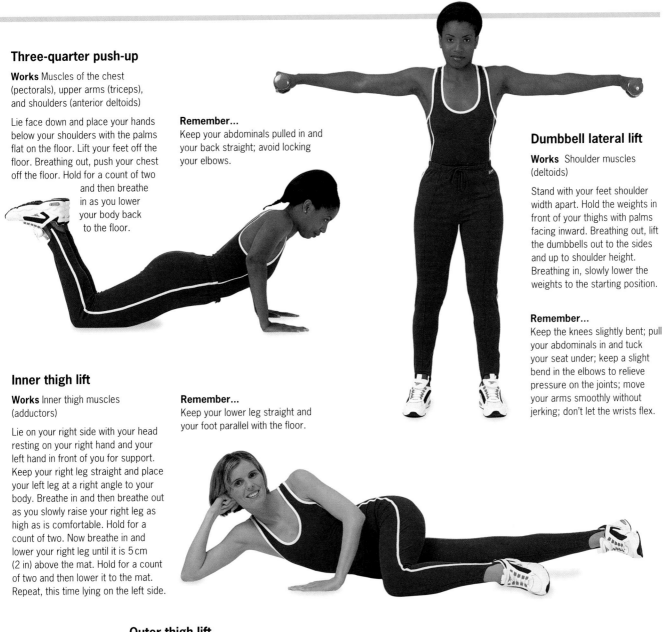

Dumbbell lateral lift

Works Shoulder muscles (deltoids)

Stand with your feet shoulder width apart. Hold the weights in front of your thighs with palms facing inward. Breathing out, lift the dumbbells out to the sides and up to shoulder height. Breathing in, slowly lower the weights to the starting position.

Remember...
Keep the knees slightly bent; pull your abdominals in and tuck your seat under; keep a slight bend in the elbows to relieve pressure on the joints; move your arms smoothly without jerking; don't let the wrists flex.

Inner thigh lift

Works Inner thigh muscles (adductors)

Lie on your right side with your head resting on your right hand and your left hand in front of you for support. Keep your right leg straight and place your left leg at a right angle to your body. Breathe in and then breathe out as you slowly raise your right leg as high as is comfortable. Hold for a count of two. Now breathe in and lower your right leg until it is 5 cm (2 in) above the mat. Hold for a count of two and then lower it to the mat. Repeat, this time lying on the left side.

Remember...
Keep your lower leg straight and your foot parallel with the floor.

Outer thigh lift

Works Outer thigh muscles (abductors)

Lie on your right side with your head resting on your right hand and your left hand on the mat in front of you for support. Bend your right knee back and keep your left leg straight. Raise your left leg as high as is comfortable. Hold the

position for a count of two. Lower your leg until it is 5 cm (2 in) above the mat. Hold the position for a count of two and then lower your leg to the mat.

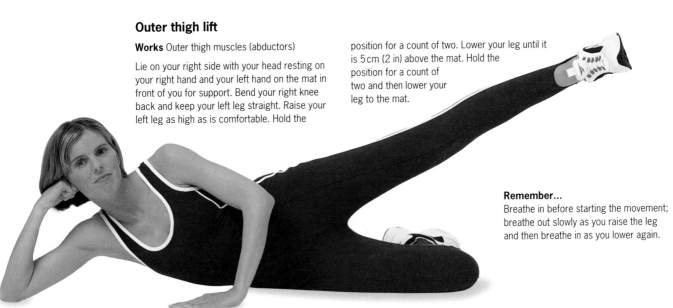

Remember...
Breathe in before starting the movement; breathe out slowly as you raise the leg and then breathe in as you lower again.

131

EXERCISE AND YOUR LIFESTYLE

Having a sedentary occupation or mobility problems resulting from age or illness can make exercise difficult to manage and lead to a decline in general health and fitness.

Many people lead a sedentary life either because their jobs offer few opportunities for physical activity or they suffer from a condition that makes regular exercise problematic. Arthritis, for example, can make weight-bearing exercise difficult and painful; as a result, many sufferers find themselves becoming increasingly inactive. Unfortunately, being sedentary can cause serious health problems.

HEALTH PROBLEMS

Sitting for long periods can lead to sagging muscles, poor posture, and sluggish circulatory and lymphatic systems; in turn, the delivery of oxygen and nutrients to the body's tissues becomes less efficient. As lymphatic functioning declines, toxic by-products begin to accumulate in the body.

Physical agility is also affected by keeping the body constantly in a flexed position. For instance, office workers who sit at a desk all day may find that their knee and hip joints gradually lose some of their range of motion because the surrounding muscles shorten. Acids also build up in muscle tissues as stress-induced tension occurs. To make matters worse, office workers may rush their meals and consume stimulants such as coffee and chocolate bars and other sugar-rich foods to pep up their flagging energy.

Poor health or illness can also create a worsening spiral of immobility, which makes both exercise and the preparation of healthful meals more difficult. These conditions in turn can lead to a lack of energy, decreasing physical fitness, and a lowering of immune function.

Just a few simple adjustments in lifestyle and environment can prevent such a scenario. The most important thing is to get moving and keep active in any way you can. The older you are, the more important it is to exercise regularly and stay active to avoid becoming overweight. Excess weight brings increased health risks, such as heart disease, stroke, and certain forms of cancer.

KEEPING ACTIVE

Lack of fitness can lead us to underestimate the body's capabilities, and in our daily routines we may come to rely too heavily on labor-saving devices. Developing an exercise habit can have a profound and positive effect upon health, enjoyment of life, and productivity at work.

A more active lifestyle can be achieved in a number of different ways, depending on circumstances. For example, you might consider the possibility of cycling to work instead of driving the car or taking a bus. Alternatively, if you leave home a little earlier, you can get off the bus or train one or two stops before your usual one and walk the rest of the way at a brisk pace.

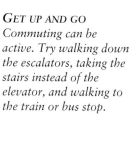

GET UP AND GO
Commuting can be active. Try walking down the escalators, taking the stairs instead of the elevator, and walking to the train or bus stop.

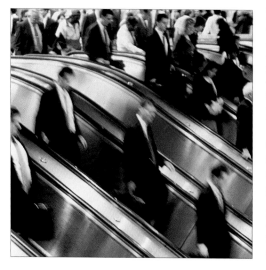

Seated Exercises

Many people spend long periods of time in a chair, either because they work in a desk-bound job or because illness makes exercise difficult. However, there are a number of exercises you can perform while seated that will improve circulation and flexibility.

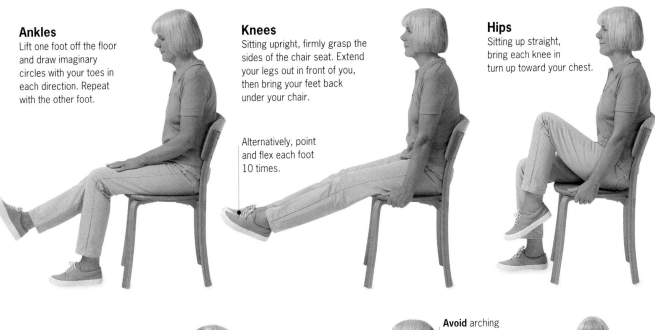

Ankles
Lift one foot off the floor and draw imaginary circles with your toes in each direction. Repeat with the other foot.

Knees
Sitting upright, firmly grasp the sides of the chair seat. Extend your legs out in front of you, then bring your feet back under your chair.

Alternatively, point and flex each foot 10 times.

Hips
Sitting up straight, bring each knee in turn up toward your chest.

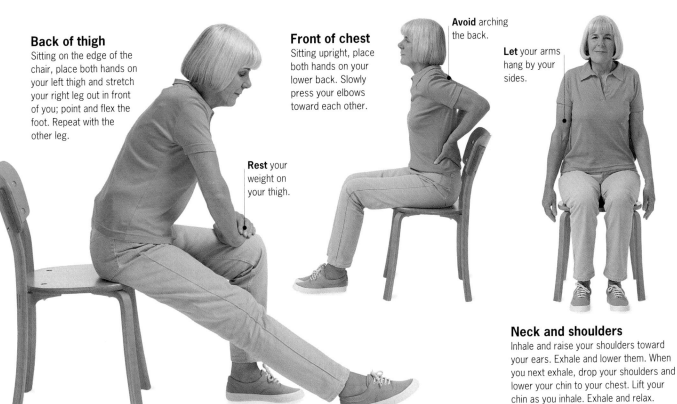

Back of thigh
Sitting on the edge of the chair, place both hands on your left thigh and stretch your right leg out in front of you; point and flex the foot. Repeat with the other leg.

Front of chest
Sitting upright, place both hands on your lower back. Slowly press your elbows toward each other.

Rest your weight on your thigh.

Avoid arching the back.

Let your arms hang by your sides.

Neck and shoulders
Inhale and raise your shoulders toward your ears. Exhale and lower them. When you next exhale, drop your shoulders and lower your chin to your chest. Lift your chin as you inhale. Exhale and relax.

If illness means you spend much of the day in a sedentary position, your muscles are likely to become stiff and sore. There are a number of gentle exercises you can do at home to improve the situation. If you have a condition such as arthritis or osteoporosis, ask your doctor or a physical therapist to suggest a program of specific movements that will suit your needs.

The most common cause of muscle pain among office workers is immobility. This problem can be avoided by taking a moment every 30 minutes to relax and by not sitting for longer than one hour at a time. Find a reason to get up and move about for 5 minutes every hour. If you can't think of anything else, get up and go for a drink of water. Not only will this get you moving, but it will also help keep you hydrated throughout the day.

If you have to read a long document, try standing and stretching your lower body while doing so. By moving around and re-aligning your body position, you will give both your body and your mind a welcome rush of blood that will stimulate all your muscles and nerve endings.

OUTSIDE ACTIVITY

It is a good idea to get outdoors for some period of time every day. One approach is to walk at least part of the way to and from work or school. Another is to go for a walk during lunchtime or a coffee break; you will be surprised at how much this activity enhances your ability to concentrate. The natural light and change of air and scenery will improve your mood and revitalize you for the rest of the day.

If age or illness means you spend a lot of time indoors, a daily walk can be an opportunity not only for exercise but also for contact with other people. Having a friend join you for a walk can also brighten up your day and boost your energy and health.

THE OFFICE GYM

With a little imagination it is possible to use many of the standard items of furniture or equipment in your office as props for a daily exercise routine. As long as the objects are fixed to the wall or floor or placed against a wall for support—a filing cabinet, for example—or so heavy that you cannot move them—a large desk, for instance—they will generally be safe enough for you to use them for support.

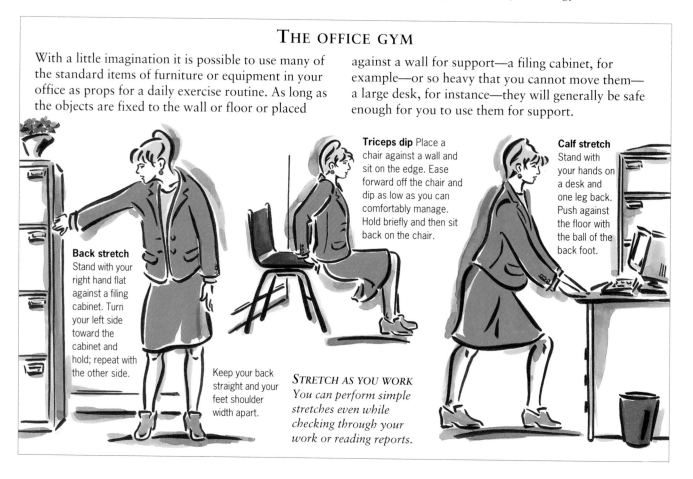

Back stretch Stand with your right hand flat against a filing cabinet. Turn your left side toward the cabinet and hold; repeat with the other side.

Triceps dip Place a chair against a wall and sit on the edge. Ease forward off the chair and dip as low as you can comfortably manage. Hold briefly and then sit back on the chair.

Keep your back straight and your feet shoulder width apart.

STRETCH AS YOU WORK You can perform simple stretches even while checking through your work or reading reports.

Calf stretch Stand with your hands on a desk and one leg back. Push against the floor with the ball of the back foot.

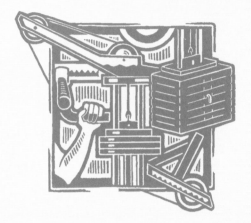

CHAPTER 8

MAKING THE MOST OF A HEALTH CLUB

Good help and instruction, a variety of facilities, and pleasant surroundings at a health club can improve your chances of sticking with an exercise program. The financial commitment you have made or the incentive of working out with others can also help sustain your interest and motivation.

CHOOSING AN EXERCISE CLUB

Once you've decided to start an exercise program, you will find it's much easier to keep it up if you feel happy and comfortable in your surroundings.

With the growing popularity of exercise as a leisure pursuit, new health clubs are opening all the time, and existing ones are updating their facilities to attract new customers. A range of choices is available in many areas, so it's worthwhile drawing up a checklist of services you would like and visiting different facilities before choosing one.

FACTORS TO CONSIDER

The first decision you must make is whether to join a private health or athletic club, a community recreation center, or a YWCA or YMCA. The main differences among the types usually relate to membership rules and fee structures, but other factors, such as individualized customer service, additional amenities, and staffing levels may also vary.

Community recreation centers and Ys usually cater to families and a broad spectrum of the public, whereas health clubs may have an air of exclusivity, which some people welcome but others find off-putting. When you visit each facility, make a point of talking to members in the gym, classes, and refreshment area for a perspective other than that of the sales representative. You may find that one place has many people whose age and background are similar to yours, which will make you feel more comfortable. You may also discover that a place is oversubscribed and is very crowded, especially in the evening or early morning hours.

Fees and membership options are important considerations. Most health clubs are privately run, either by an individual owner or a larger organization, and tend to be more expensive. When you become a member, you generally pay a one-time joining fee and then monthly or annual dues, and you can use the facilities as often as you like. Some people like the commitment that this system involves, as well as the fact that the more often you exercise, the more value you will get for your money.

Community centers are often subsidized by a town or other regional authority. Fee structures tend to be more reasonable and flexible, especially for families; you may be able to pay just for attending classes or buy a pass that allows you to use all facilities a certain number of within a specified period. If you plan to exercise only once or twice a week, a community center may be a more cost-effective choice.

HISTORY OF THE GYMNASIUM

The word *gymnasium* comes from the ancient Greek verb *gumnazein*, meaning "to exercise naked." Exercises were originally performed without weights and were designed to enhance balance, strength, and coordination. Although the practice is most closely associated with Greece, the ancient Persians, Romans, Indians, and Chinese also exercised in this way. Modern gymnastics evolved from calisthenics (from the Greek word *kallos*, for "beauty" and *sthenos*, for "grace"), which developed in the 1800s in Germany and Sweden. Weights were introduced to prepare the body for gymnastic events. Today most people use gymnasiums to stay fit rather than to prepare for gymnastic competitions.

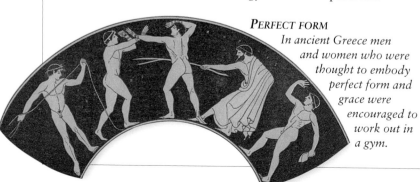

PERFECT FORM
In ancient Greece men and women who were thought to embody perfect form and grace were encouraged to work out in a gym.

Club location

The location of a club or center is also an important consideration, depending on the time of day that you plan to exercise. If you intend to work out during your lunch break or immediately before or after work, for example, it would be best to choose a club that is close to your workplace. On the other hand, if you plan to exercise later in the evening or on weekends or if you have free time during the day, you might prefer to join a health club that is within a reasonable distance of your home.

You should also check on the club's hours, which can vary widely, and make sure that the one you choose is open at times that fit in with your lifestyle.

If you are going to drive to your place of exercise, parking facilities may also influence your decision. Check that there is a sufficient number of parking spaces for the members actively using the club and that lighting and other security aspects are adequate. If you use public transportation, look for a health club that is close to a bus or train route. Alternatively, consider a club within walking or cycling distance, which offers an ideal way to warm up before your exercise session.

Visiting the facilities

Most health clubs and community centers are listed in local newspapers and the telephone directory, but advertising alone is not a reliable way to choose a facility. You should elicit comments from exercisers you know. If a club has been highly recommended by one of your friends, it's well worth a visit. Health clubs normally offer a tour of their facilities, and it is advisable to make

---

CHOOSING A HEALTH CLUB

When looking for a suitable exercise facility, you should draw up a list of the health clubs or community centers that match your particular needs and lifestyle. Before you make your final decision, arrange to look around the premises and feel free to ask the staff questions. The tour should include a visit to the changing rooms, which should be clean, fresh smelling, well ventilated, and have an adequate number of showers. These often provide a good indication of the general standards of the club.

Costs
Inquire about a club's fee structure to help you decide whether to buy a membership or pay per visit.

Safety guidelines
Information on the safe use of equipment and other facilities should be prominently displayed.

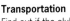

Qualifications
Staff qualifications, including first aid certificates, should be clearly on view in the reception area.

Children's facilities
If you are buying a family membership, find out if child care is available and what facilities children may use.

Gym equipment
Check that there is a range of equipment, that it is well maintained, and that it is sufficient for the number of members.

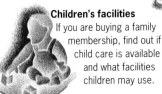

Courses
Make sure that the classes available will suit your current needs and also accommodate your future aspirations.

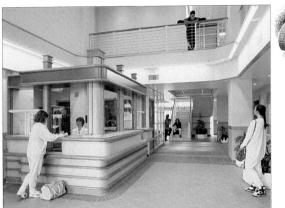

Transportation
Find out if the club or center is close to main bus or train routes and if there are adequate services.

Parking facilities
Make sure that there are enough parking spaces at busy times and that the parking area is well lit for dark evenings.

Opening hours
Check that the facilities you want to use will be available at the times you are most likely to need them and are not overcrowded during those periods.

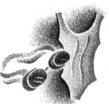

Additional services
Ask whether extra facilities are available, such as a swimming pool, sauna, or massage services.

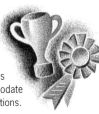

137

ON-SITE CHILD CARE
Many health clubs offer child care for members' children. Parents with young children often find it convenient to exercise during the day and take advantage of this facility. Such a nursery should be staffed by qualified personnel and have adequate space and equipment.

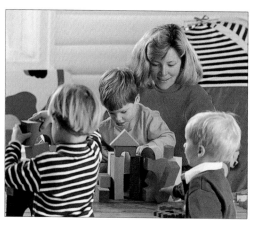

full use of this opportunity to ask as many questions as you can. A staff member should also spend time with you to discuss your fitness goals and motivation for starting a program.

Try not to feel intimidated by the fitness of members or complexity of equipment you see during a tour. A good health club will make sure that you are shown how to use each piece of equipment and understand which muscle groups it is designed to exercise before you begin your training program. Find out also if the instruction is individualized or is given in a class setting.

You may be required to have a fitness assessment done so that an instructor can draw up a training program for you. These assessments can vary considerably from one facility to another, but their main purpose is to establish your current level of cardiovascular health, as well as strength and flexibility, and to ensure that any training regimen arranged for you will suit your particular requirements and abilities. An assessment also provides a record of your initial fitness level so you can gauge your progress over the course of the program.

You should also assure yourself that the staff members are suitably qualified. Many health clubs put the certificates of their instructors on display near the reception desk. These should include certification in aerobics (see page 150) and/or other forms of exercise plus first aid. If these qualifications are not evident, make a point of asking about them during your initial tour.

The range of equipment that health clubs provide varies considerably. A trainer will tailor fitness programs according to the facilities available. You may prefer to use a variety of exercise machines, however, so check that the place has everything you are

likely to need. These might include jogging or walking treadmills, cross-country ski machines, rowing machines, stationary bikes, strength-building apparatus, multi-gyms, and free-standing weights.

Every club should have guidelines for the safe use of their facilities and equipment. These should be explained to you during your initial assessment or induction and be available in either leaflet format or as posters prominently displayed on the walls, which you can inspect when necessary.

If you plan to take classes in such activities as aerobics, t'ai chi, or yoga, make sure the club offers a variety of them, that they cater to all levels of ability, and that they are given at times of the day that suit you.

Additional facilities

Many health clubs provide help with weight management. If losing weight is one goal of your exercise program, it is worthwhile joining a club that recognizes the close link between activity and nutrition and has staff members qualified to offer you sound and practical dietary advice.

A number of clubs include such amenities as a sauna, Jacuzzi, and/or steam room, which provide a good way to recover from a grueling exercise session or to help you unwind after a stressful day at work.

Tanning beds are also available at some health clubs but should be used with caution because excessive use can lead to skin damage, premature aging, and an increased risk of skin cancer. A good health club will have safety guidelines clearly displayed and will offer you practical advice on their use.

Some health clubs also offer ancillary services, which might include massage therapy, hairdressing, and skin care, at extra cost. Many people find this arrangement both convenient and time-saving.

> **CAUTION**
> *Tanning beds should always be used with care. They should be avoided altogether if you:*
> ► *are under age 16.*
> ► *are prone to sunburn.*
> ► *have a history of skin cancer in the family.*
> ► *have a lot of freckles or moles.*

GETTING STARTED

Your first session at a gym can be intimidating, but if you are clear about your goals and your needs, you will be able to get the most out of the instructors and facilities.

Once you have decided which health club you will join, the next step is to get yourself ready for action. Most health clubs will give you a fitness assessment, introduce you to the machines, and help you design a training program, but only you can know exactly what it is you want to achieve.

It is important to give this careful thought before your introduction so you can explain your personal goals and ambitions to the fitness instructor (see page 59). The instructor can then tailor your program to your specific needs rather than making you follow a general routine that may be given to all new members. Keeping your goals in mind will help you to stay focused and motivated throughout your time at the club.

TRAINING REGIMEN

Unless you establish clear goals, it is very likely that you will abandon your fitness regimen prematurely. On the other hand, according to research conducted by an American exercise psychologist, Dr. Rod Dishman, there is a significant increase in frequency, intensity, duration, and perseverance in fitness regimens if they are started and maintained for clearly understood and personal reasons.

Other important issues to consider are regularity and consistency. It is better not to skip any sessions unless you are ill. You should also aim to set yourself a new target at each workout. Given the correct exercise stimulus, your body will soon adapt to the routine and become stronger, more supple, and more aerobically fit. At the same time, make any changes to your lifestyle that will bolster your fitness program. Integrating regular exercise with a healthy diet, adequate sleep, and reasonable working routines and social activities will achieve the greatest long-term results.

PLANNING YOUR ROUTINE

Your gym fitness adviser will help you plan a routine that takes into account your goals, but as a general rule, you will have to establish one that you can perform for at least 20 minutes three times a week. Try to include both cardiovascular training (exercise that increases your heart rate for at least 12 minutes at a time) and resistance work (strength exercises) in your regimen. Your cardiovascular ability will be limited if your muscles are not strong enough to sustain exercise, and similarly, your strength will be limited if you don't have sufficient stamina to keep you going throughout the session.

Most people begin their workout with cardiovascular training because it does not deplete energy reserves. Attempting cardiovascular exercise at the end of your routine may prove difficult because a resistance workout may already have worn you out.

A positive approach
It is important to keep a positive attitude toward exercise classes. Decide on clear and realistic long-term fitness targets and make up your mind to see the course through. Research shows that the highest dropout rate from fitness classes occurs in the first two months among people who are unclear about their goals and have become dispirited because they do not feel they are making good progress.

COMBINATION EXERCISE

A rowing machine works all the major muscle groups at the same time and improves both strength and aerobic fitness. Rowing works the muscles and joints in the legs and back while giving the arms a resistance workout, and the overall action offers good cardiovascular exercise.

INCREASED GAIN
The resistance can be increased on a rowing machine to provide a harder workout.

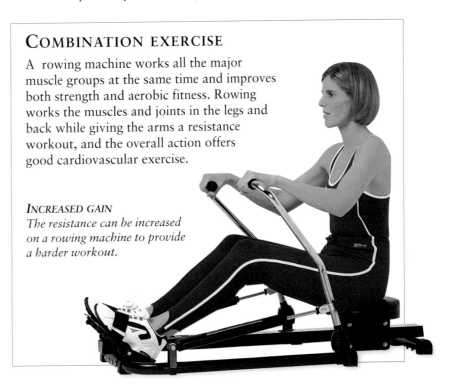

CARDIOVASCULAR TRAINING
Options for cardiovascular training at a gym usually include aerobic, step, and circuit training classes, and running, rowing, cycling, skiing, and step machines. When starting a cardiovascular program, it is worth trying out the low-impact alternatives as your first move. Too much unaccustomed impact through excessive jumping, bouncing, or jogging is a primary cause of many limb disorders and injuries such as shin splints. Fortunately, most machines in

---

THE GYM: A BEGINNER'S GUIDE

Once you have joined a gym, you can obtain full benefit from it by asking questions about the use of equipment and any of the classes and amenities offered. If you are intimidated about using some of the facilities, you may give up on your exercise program simply because you feel uncomfortable in the surroundings. Take time to try out all the various pieces of equipment and classes to see which ones best meet your needs. The more variety you put into your routine, the more motivated you are likely to become.

1. Determine your goals
Decide what you want to achieve at the gym. Do you want to improve your overall aerobic fitness and muscle tone, or are you looking to strengthen an injured or weakened muscle group?

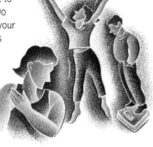

2. Visit the gym Check out the center, examine its facilities, and have a fitness assessment done. Discuss your fitness goals with an instructor and ask about the different classes and types of exercise equipment available that would suit your specific needs.

3. Decide how often you can visit
Establish a basic plan for visiting the gym. You can build up the frequency and intensity of your exercise sessions gradually to avoid overstressing your body, but you should start with a minimal commitment of 20 minutes of exercise three times a week.

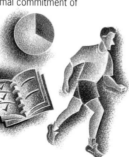

4. Plan your routine at the gym
Your particular routine should reflect the specific goals you have established, but as a general rule, most people should include in each session both aerobic activities for at least 12 minutes, to increase heart and breathing rates, and resistance exercises that work specific muscle groups.

5. Begin with cardiovascular exercise
If you are planning a 20-minute session, devote 15 minutes to cardiovascular exercise. Options include aerobic exercises and running, cycling, and rowing machines. Include muscle-building exercises in your routine as well.

7. Relax and unwind
Remember that your visit should be fun; take advantage of the varied facilities offered. For example, try a relaxing massage or a sauna to soothe and relax tired muscles.

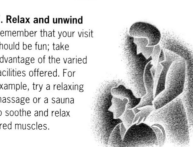

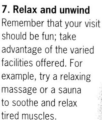

6. Decide on the type of resistance work
Resistance training options include weight machines and free weights, as well as aqua aerobics and body sculpting. Your fitness assessment will help you focus on the muscle groups that need the most attention. In addition to boosting the strength and endurance of muscles, resistance exercises can improve appearance by making muscles firmer and more clearly defined.

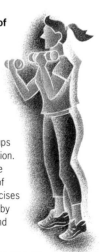

clubs are low impact by design (an exception is the treadmill, but even this provides more cushioning for the limbs than running on roads or pavement).

In aerobics classes the format and style should vary according to the fitness levels of the class members. A competent teacher will be able to adapt most movements from low to high impact and alter the intensity to suit the fitness of all the participants.

Ideally, the activities in a class should be varied on a regular basis. For a change you could also attend two or three different types of classes (see page 149). In addition to reducing the potential for boredom and reducing the risk of repetitive-use injuries, variety will create the necessary stimulus for constant adaptation by the body and ensure that certain muscle groups are not overexercised while others are neglected.

FLEXIBILITY TRAINING

Although most exercise equipment is designed primarily for developing muscles and/or cardiovascular fitness, a few machines, such as the cross-country skiing machine, also work on flexibility. Aerobics, aqua aerobics, and body sculpting classes help develop suppleness as well. And many clubs offer yoga classes, which can be particularly helpful in this regard. A major focus in yoga is the gradual stretching out of all muscles to attain maximum flexibility.

MUSCULAR TRAINING

Strength training primarily involves the use of weight machines, although aqua aerobics and body sculpting classes also improve the strength of specific muscles. You should aim to develop a well-balanced routine. Muscles operate in pairs across most joints to provide balance and protection, so it is important that equal strength is maintained in each pair. An imbalance in muscle pairs is a common underlying cause of joint pain; neck problems may be the result of weak upper back and shoulder muscles, for example. A balanced routine will include an exercise for each muscle of the pair, such as chest with upper back muscles, shoulders with middle back muscles, abdominals with lower back, biceps with triceps, thighs with hamstrings, and calf muscles with shins.

It is not advisable to condition only the muscles of the lower body—for example, through step routines or running—while neglecting the upper portion. For optimal conditioning, it is best to select machines that utilize both upper and lower body function. The use of either a rowing machine or a cross-country skiing machine will accomplish this. What's more, greater initial gains can be made from exercising the upper body, and these gains may quickly be noticed in everyday life. For instance, you may soon find you're able to lift shopping bags or a young child without straining.

Correct exercise technique

For effective and safe exercising, you must use the correct technique for each exercise and take extra care when you are beginning to feel tired. Deviating from correct technique can result in injury to a muscle or the connective tissue in a joint. For example, lifting a weight without proper control threatens the integrity of other muscles or joint structures that try to cope with a sudden load they are not prepared for or do not have the strength to handle. It also defeats the purpose because the muscles originally targeted will not be exercised properly.

MR. UNIVERSE

The man who became known as the Father of Modern Bodybuilding was Oscar Heidenstam (1911–1991). His career in bodybuilding began when he became the first British bodybuilder to win the Mr. Europe contest in 1939.

An exemplary sportsman, Heidenstam was internationally acknowledged as the foremost ambassador and expert in bodybuilding during its formative years. He became the publisher of the world's longest established physical culture magazine, *Health and Strength*, which was founded in 1898. Continuing his close links with the sport, in 1956 Heidenstam organized the most famous and long-standing world bodybuilding contest, Mr. Universe.

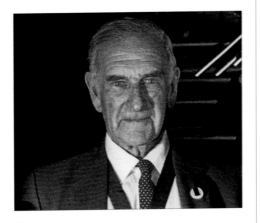

OSCAR HEIDENSTAM
A modest humanitarian, Oscar Heidenstam was famed for his motivational and inspirational skills and lived by his credo, "Do good by stealth and blush to find it known."

USING EQUIPMENT

Although some people think of exercise and weight-training paraphernalia as the domain of the serious athlete, many pieces of equipment offer benefits for the more moderate exerciser.

The equipment available in a gym can be grouped into two main categories: cardiovascular—used to strengthen the heart, lungs, and circulation—and resistance—used to strengthen muscles. Understanding how to use the equipment and deciding which pieces best meet your needs are integral to an exercise plan.

CARDIOVASCULAR EQUIPMENT
Cardiovascular machines not only improve overall fitness levels but also provide a good warm-up exercise prior to a session on resistance machines. They include devices like treadmills, rowing machines, step machines, aerobic bikes, and cross-country skiing simulators. These different types of equipment will also tone specific muscle groups. For example, step and cycling machines tone the leg muscles, while rowing and skiing machines provide all-over muscle toning.

RESISTANCE EQUIPMENT
Whether you use exercise machines, free weights, elastic bands, or your own body weight for resistance training, this is the most effective form of exercise for enhancing muscular strength, size, and power. Most gyms and health clubs have a range of resistance apparatus available; the type that a person selects is often determined by personal preference. Some people enjoy the ease of using machines and the fact that they require a minimum of training to master. Machines are also easy to adjust, so you can make steady progress.

FREE WEIGHTS VERSUS MACHINES

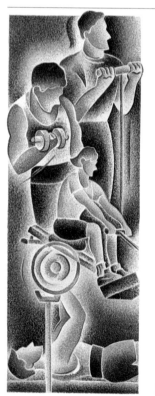

There are advantages and disadvantages to both free weights and machines. Before you commit yourself to buying a piece of resistance exercise equipment, weigh such factors as the cost, available space, ease of use, and your exercise goals.

FREE WEIGHTS	MACHINES
They are relatively inexpensive.	They are expensive.
They need accurate technique to be effective.	They are easy to use.
They take up minimal space.	They take up substantial space.
Using heavier weights may require help from a partner.	Heavier weights are easily controlled.
Changing weight plates can be time-consuming.	Increasing the degree of resistance is a quick process.
It is easy to target specific muscles.	They are best when used to work muscle groups.
They are good for toning and firming muscles.	They are best for building strength and bulk.
They need minimal maintenance.	They need regular maintenance.
They work support muscles that aid good posture.	They work support muscles less.
They are suitable for people of all builds.	Some are best for average builds only.

Other people prefer free weights because they provide a greater range of movement, thus giving individuals more control over which muscles they develop and how they develop them. (Resistance machines can be modified, however, to help you focus on certain muscle groups.) Whichever form of resistance training you choose, you must always use correct technique to exercise safely. If you have any doubts about how to use a particular piece of equipment, ask an instructor to demonstrate it for you.

Pin-selected weight stack

A pin-selected weight stack is common to many types of resistance machines. It is a stack of weight plates with a central rod running through them, which allows for lifting various weights. Make sure the machine you are using has adjustable training positions so you can alter it to fit your body size and shape. A major advantage of resistance machines is the ease with which each movement can be learned. You will also quickly recognize how the working muscles should feel when exercising properly, so you obtain maximum benefits with minimum risk.

Free weights

Free weights can be either dumbbells, which are available in a range of fixed sizes, or barbells (see page 123), which can be loaded with discs of varying weights. These discs are attached to each end of the bar and can be built up to total any weight desired.

In addition to working the main muscle groups, free weights also utilize many of the minor fixating (support) muscles that help to control, balance, and stabilize the body during resistance exercises. They thus exercise the body in a more natural way than is possible with exercise machines and also enhance overall muscle strength.

The main disadvantage of free weights is that a high degree of skill is needed to use them in a safe and controlled way and to ensure that the main muscle groups perform the lion's share of the work. Without sufficiently developed neuromuscular control, it is difficult to lift free weights correctly. As a consequence, excess stress may be placed on the back or on a joint or muscle that is too weak to cope with it, thus increasing the risk of serious injury. Like all new skills, controlling free weights should be learned properly from a skilled instructor.

MACHINE MONITORS

Many exercise machines have computerized gauges that enable you to check your performance. The readouts from these machines can help you to fine-tune your fitness routine for optimum benefits. On some machines the computation may include:

▶ *intensity of exercise*
▶ *duration of exercise*
▶ *distance traveled*
▶ *speed traveled*
▶ *heart rate*
▶ *total calories used during the session*
▶ *lung capacity*
▶ *changes in blood pressure*
▶ *recovery rate*

SIMPLE RESISTANCE EQUIPMENT

You don't need to use complicated machinery in the gym to improve your strength. There are some gym exercises—such as triceps dips—that involve the use of a workout bench and your body weight alone to condition and tone the muscles.

Many gym goers also make use of simple props for resistance exercises. The most common nonweight props are lengths of rubber tubing or elastic bands of varying degrees of resistance. These can be pulled between the hands, for example, or attached to a foot and stretched. Because the resistance comes from stretching the rubber rather than from the force of gravity acting upon a weight, imaginative exercisers can use these props to devise virtually any kind of resistance movement they choose. The effect of using an elastic band is similar to that of some resistance machines. Looking at how particular machines work can help you devise elastic band exercises.

Also simple and widely used are wrist and ankle weights, which increase the load that the arms and legs have to bear when performing resistance exercises. They can also be used during cardiovascular workouts like aerobic sessions or walking. Some ankle weights contain individual weight bags to permit varying the load according to the type of exercise being done and increase it as muscular strength improves.

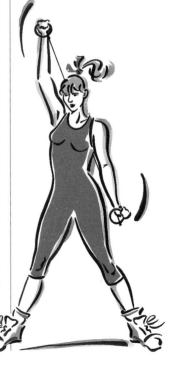

ELASTIC BANDS
Like free weights, elastic bands allow a natural range of movement and can exercise both the assisting and stabilizing muscles, as well as the major muscle groups.

Resistance Work

The resistance machines shown here are typical of the ones found in most gyms for developing muscular strength and endurance. A trainer can advise you about the amount of resistance and number of repetitions you need to attain your fitness goals.

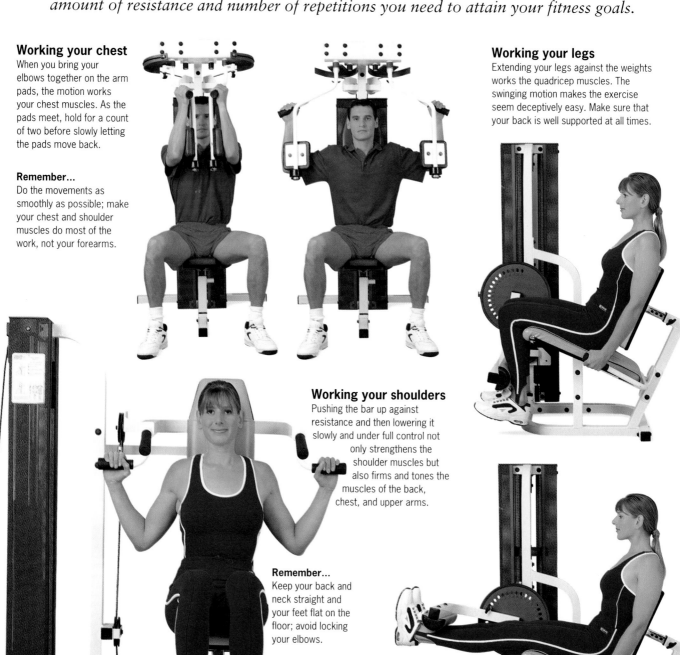

Working your chest
When you bring your elbows together on the arm pads, the motion works your chest muscles. As the pads meet, hold for a count of two before slowly letting the pads move back.

Remember...
Do the movements as smoothly as possible; make your chest and shoulder muscles do most of the work, not your forearms.

Working your legs
Extending your legs against the weights works the quadricep muscles. The swinging motion makes the exercise seem deceptively easy. Make sure that your back is well supported at all times.

Working your shoulders
Pushing the bar up against resistance and then lowering it slowly and under full control not only strengthens the shoulder muscles but also firms and tones the muscles of the back, chest, and upper arms.

Remember...
Keep your back and neck straight and your feet flat on the floor; avoid locking your elbows.

Remember...
Keep your movements flowing; let your legs do the work, not your back, and try not to favor one leg over the other; keep the head and neck relaxed.

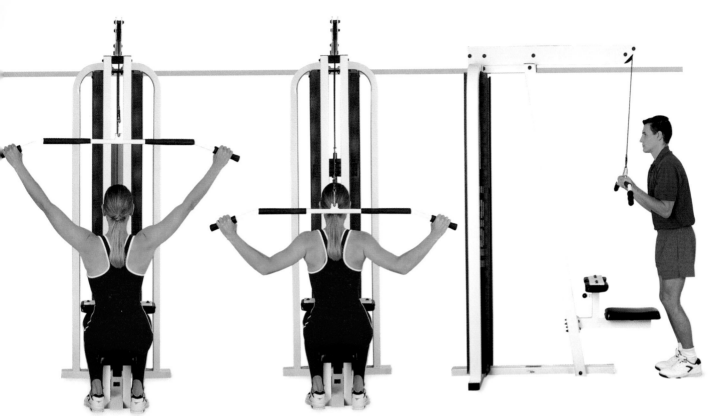

Working your back
To work the muscles of the arms, shoulders, and back, pull down the bar on a high pulley from above your head to behind it. Don't pull the bar too low behind you, as this will overstretch the muscles.

Remember...
Keep your wrists straight; adjust the bar above the seat to secure your knees; keep your knees in line with your feet and your feet flat on the floor; hold your abdominal muscles in and keep your back straight.

Working your arms
Pull down on the weighted bar until it is about chest height, then raise and lower the bar, working your forearms below the elbow.

Remember...
Keep your movements fluid; do not jerk your arms; keep your back straight and your feet flat on the floor.

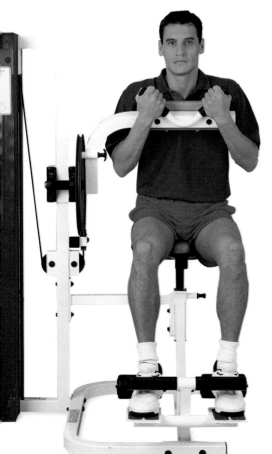

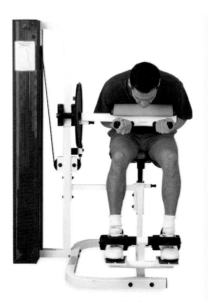

Working your abdominals
Lowering your torso slowly against resistance strengthens the abdominal muscles and works the muscles of the lower back. Keep your abdominal muscles tight and breathe out as you lean forward.

Remember...
Keep your neck and spine in line and make sure your feet are secured and held flat against the foot rest.

FOR BEST RESULTS
After completing the last set of resistance exercises, start to perform cool-down activities as soon as possible. Choose a full-body aerobic activity to work all muscles that have been used in the resistance workout.

Right after cooling down is the ideal time to enhance your flexibility because your muscles are at their most elastic. Permanent improvements in a muscle's mobility can be made with appropriate stretches.

Stretch imbalanced muscles to increase your range of motion at the joint, using the same stretches as those used in the warm-up but more extensively. When you reach the point of initial stretch sensation, hold the position for 20 to 30 seconds or even a minute or more if comfortable in the position.

Muscle Problems

Although the benefits of keeping fit outweigh any negative aspects, there may be times when you push yourself too hard and experience aches, cramps, or stitches. Given here are simple steps you can take to relieve these common problems.

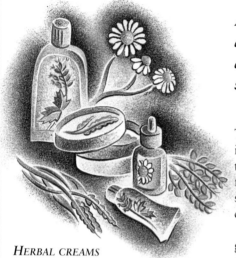

HERBAL CREAMS
You can often avoid muscle soreness or cramps by applying a warming ointment or cream that contains an herb like wintergreen before exercising.

The sensation of pain caused by injury, overexercising, incorrect technique, or other factors generally falls into three categories: instant, sharp, and debilitating; nagging and chronic; and short-term.

Sudden sharp, debilitating pain generally signifies a serious injury, which you should not attempt to treat yourself but instead seek medical advice right away.

Chronic, or long-term, pain usually indicates a structural weakness of the body, joint inflammation, minor muscle tears, or stiff and imbalanced muscles, any of which you may be able to treat yourself. The problem will usually be resolved with a period of rest, but if the pain continues, you should seek medical help.

Short-term pain that comes on during or shortly after exercise and gradually eases after a few hours is usually caused by intense fatigue and momentary muscle failure. It is not generally a serious problem.

RELIEVING MUSCLE CRAMP

A cramp is characterized by very painful and strong localized muscle contractions. It usually occurs after a sustained period of exercise that involves strenuous muscular work, such as a hard game of soccer, an intense aerobic workout, or a long run. A cramp is primarily caused by

an imbalance of two minerals—sodium and potassium—which regulate the electrical impulses that make the muscles work. Normally these minerals interact alternately to contract and relax muscles, but when an imbalance occurs, the muscles still contract but then are not able to relax immediately afterward. A

cramp can be relieved at once by massaging and stretching the affected muscles as far as possible to relax them. For most cramps you can do this for yourself or you can ask an exercise companion to do it for you. As a preventive measure, make sure you drink some fluid prior to and during exercise.

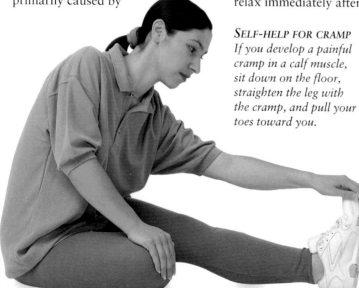

SELF-HELP FOR CRAMP
If you develop a painful cramp in a calf muscle, sit down on the floor, straighten the leg with the cramp, and pull your toes toward you.

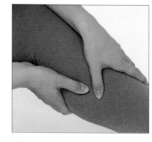

APPLY PRESSURE
To help relieve the pain of a muscle cramp, press deeply into the center of the painful area with your thumbs while you continue to stretch the muscle.

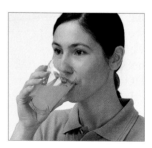

SALT AS A SOLUTION
To restore your mineral balance, add a teaspoon of salt to a glass of water or fruit juice and sip the liquid slowly; do not gulp it.

RELIEVING A STITCH

A stitch is a dull, cramplike ache, normally experienced on one side of the abdominal muscles. The underlying cause of a stitch is not known for sure, but it is thought to result from a spasm of the diaphragm muscle or localized fatigue of the muscles that stabilize the hip and trunk. A stitch usually occurs when athletes are out of shape or are pushing themselves too hard—for example, by attempting speeds greater than they are normally accustomed to—or have not thoroughly warmed up before starting their exercise routine.

A stitch may also be a consequence of exercising too soon after eating a big meal or drinking large amounts of fluid. This happens because the body diverts extra blood to the internal organs to deal with the digestive processes, thus sending insufficient oxygen to the muscles to meet the extra demands imposed by exercise.

If a stitch develops, ease down on the intensity of the exercise and take deep breaths, holding each breath for as long as is comfortable before exhaling slowly. If the stitch becomes too painful, you should stop exercising and slowly bend forward from the waist to flex the trunk, at the same time continuing to breathe deeply and slowly.

To reduce the risk of developing a stitch, you should wait a minimum of two hours between eating a big meal and starting exercise. Develop a regular breathing pattern to match your stride rate and concentrate on good technique; aim to keep your hips level and try not to overstride.

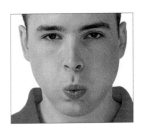

CONTROL AIR FLOW
To help control your breathing rate when suffering from a sudden stitch, make your mouth into a small circle as you slowly breathe out.

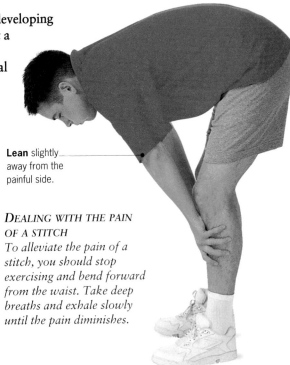

Lean slightly away from the painful side.

DEALING WITH THE PAIN OF A STITCH
To alleviate the pain of a stitch, you should stop exercising and bend forward from the waist. Take deep breaths and exhale slowly until the pain diminishes.

RELIEVING MUSCLE SORENESS

Muscle aches 24 to 48 hours after exercising are very common and are usually part of the process of physical adaptation as your body adjusts to the demands of exercise. They are often a positive sign, indicating that your muscles are expanding to cope with the increased workload you are placing on them. This belated feeling of pain is called delayed onset muscle soreness, or DOMS for short (see page 77).

If muscle soreness develops after exercise, it can be greatly eased by stretching the affected areas, carrying out a series of light activities to flex the muscles, or having a massage to soothe away the tension within the muscle fibers. A warm bath that has been run through an herbal bath bag containing such analgesic herbs as rosemary can also help to soothe the pain of sore muscles. Alternatively, a few drops of soothing essential oils, such as chamomile or marjoram, can be added to the bathwater.

Muscle pain is not an inevitable consequence of exercise, however. DOMS can be completely avoided as a rule by making sure that your exercise is not too intense for your level of fitness and by carrying out a thorough regimen of warm-up exercises before each workout and a cool-down routine afterward. The warm-up and cool-down periods should include stretches to warm, loosen, and oxygenate those muscles that do most of the work.

HERBAL RELIEF
Tie an herbal bag under the faucet so that the flowing water will release the soothing ingredients. Both thyme and rosemary have relaxing and pain-relieving properties that ease aching muscles.

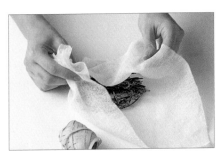

MAKING AN HERBAL BATH BAG
Lay sprigs of thyme and rosemary on a square of muslin, draw the corners of the fabric together, and tie the bundle with a piece of string or ribbon.

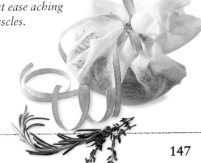

EXERCISE CLASSES

There are many different types of exercise classes, each designed to meet a particular goal or standard of fitness. You should be able to find one that meets your requirements.

Some exercise organizations cater to many different fitness levels by scheduling a variety of classes at various times of the day. Others offer a smaller number of classes aimed at a broader range of abilities. Ask for a brochure or leaflet that explains what is offered and, if necessary, request more information about a class or try it out before joining.

The facilities where classes are given can vary considerably. Some health clubs have exercise studios with a specially built wooden floor, mirrors, and a built-in sound system. In other cases, a recreation hall, dance studio, or school gymnasium, plus a cassette player for the music, may serve the purpose. The quality of a class does not depend on the sophistication of the facilities, however, because a good teacher can create a great atmosphere in the most basic setting. If a class is well attended, it usually reflects the ability of the instructor to inspire students.

PREPARATION FOR AN EXERCISE CLASS

Before attending an exercise class for the first time, there are some important factors to consider. To avoid foot injuries and blisters, you need a well-fitting and supportive pair of cross-training shoes and heavy seamless sports socks. To allow for easy, unconstrained movement, you should choose clothes that are either loose or stretchable. Wearing two or three layers is a good idea because you can remove clothing as you become warmer during the class. Also, carry a bottle of water with you and take frequent sips throughout the class.

Speak to the instructor before you start and mention that this is your first time. He or she may offer some tips on how to adapt certain exercises to make them easier for you or instruct you to stop if you become too fatigued. Always inform a teacher of any medical conditions you have.

WARMING UP
The grapevine is a popular warm-up exercise used in many fitness classes. You can also incorporate it into your personal exercise program. The grapevine is best done to music; the faster the tempo, the more effective it is at warming muscles.

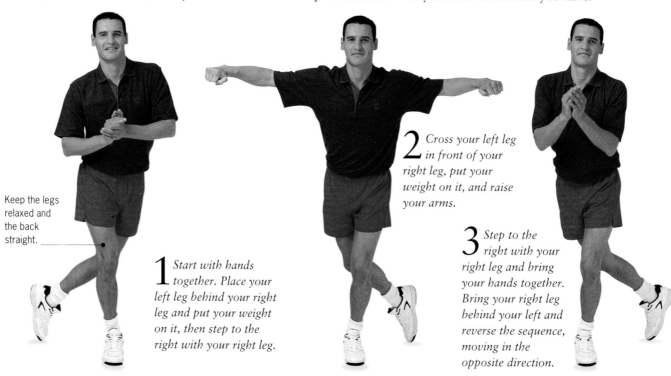

Keep the legs relaxed and the back straight.

1 *Start with hands together. Place your left leg behind your right leg and put your weight on it, then step to the right with your right leg.*

2 *Cross your left leg in front of your right leg, put your weight on it, and raise your arms.*

3 *Step to the right with your right leg and bring your hands together. Bring your right leg behind your left and reverse the sequence, moving in the opposite direction.*

148

COMPONENTS OF AN EXERCISE CLASS

A good exercise class includes a number of components, each of which will vary in length according to the type of class and the ability level of the participants.

Warm-up

A workout starts with a warm-up that lasts for at least 5 minutes. It involves rhythmical movements of the larger muscle groups that start slowly and gradually build up in pace and intensity. These prepare the body for the exercises to come by loosening the joints, raising the heart rate and respiration, and increasing the flow of blood to oxygenate and warm the muscles and make them more elastic. A warm-up should also include static stretches, each held for about 10 seconds.

Cardiovascular, or aerobic, section

Aerobic exercises increase general fitness by improving the strength and efficiency of the heart and lungs. They may be either low or high in intensity, depending on the type of class and its duration. Low-intensity movements include knee lifts and marching. Examples of high-intensity movements are jogging and high kicks.

Some classes are designated as low impact or high impact, which should not be confused with high and low intensity. The term *low impact* indicates that one foot stays in contact with the floor at all times, thus limiting the impact on the joints. A high-impact movement involves jumping, during which the weight of the body is in the air for a short duration. Low-impact moves are especially suitable for older people and those with joint disorders, but anyone can realize a good workout with them.

Muscular toning section

These exercises, which not only increase the strength of muscles but also improve body shape and make everyday tasks easier, may be included as part of an aerobics class or may be the major emphasis of a session. They are done using body weight alone or with resistance equipment, such as ankle weights, hand weights, or rubber bands.

Stretching section

The stretching section at the end of any exercise class is important and should not be skipped. Static stretches, involving the major muscle groups and held for 10 to 30 seconds, can reduce muscular soreness and tension after exercise and increase the range of movement of both joints and muscles.

TYPES OF EXERCISE CLASSES

A wide range of exercise classes is available. Some concentrate mainly on cardiovascular fitness, whereas others aim to increase the size, tone, and definition of muscles.

Aerobics

Any aerobics class includes the elements of muscular toning and stretches but puts most of the emphasis on aerobic, or cardiovascular, exercise. In order to maintain the pulse rate within the training zone, a series of energetic movements is performed for at least 20 and up to 50 minutes using a variety of foot and arm patterns, usually in combinations that form routines.

Dance aerobics

Following a format similar to that of standard aerobics classes, dance aerobics incorporate disco dance movements into the

continued on page 152

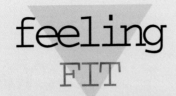

feeling
FIT

NAME				
DATE	PROGRAM	FREQUENCY	INTENSITY	TIME
1/11	Muscle toner	2 x weekly	Low	6:30pm
EXERCISE	MAX WEIGHT	SETS & REP	SEAT NO.	TIME (min)
Warm-up				10–15
Leg press	2 blocks	3 x 12–15	7	
Leg curl	1 block	2 x 10–12	7	
Chest press	1 block	3 x 12–15	3	
Shoulder press	1 block	3 x 12–15	4	
Lateral pull-down	3 blocks	2 x 10–12	4	
Seated curl	1 block	3 x 12–15	2	
ADDITIONAL INSTRUCTOR ADVICE/ COMMENTS				

TRAINING SCHEDULE
When you join a gym, a fitness instructor should fill out a training schedule for your personal optimum workout and review it following a progress assessment, usually after a few weeks. This ensures that your training is always tailored to your needs.

The Aerobics Instructor

A good aerobics class has an instructor who is qualified, experienced, and able to motivate the class. It doesn't matter whether the class is held in a modern exercise studio or a church hall, as long as it suits your individual needs.

POWER BOOST
Wearing wrist and ankle weights or holding dumbbells while doing aerobics can help improve muscle tone.

Origins

Aerobic dancing originated in the United States in the 1970s and is credited to Jackie Sorenson, an exercise specialist and dancer. She aimed to make keeping fit more fun by combining exercises for stamina and stretches for suppleness with a background of music. The original high-impact aerobics and the concept of "no pain, no gain" have now been replaced with healthier forms, such as low-impact step aerobics.

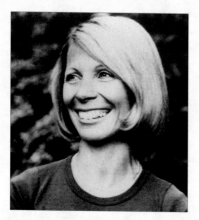

FITNESS BOOM
The aerobic dance classes devised by Jackie Sorenson quickly became an integral part of the exercise boom of the 1980s.

Joining an aerobics class can be fun as well as good for health. Much of the benefit derived will depend on how skillful the teacher is at building the pace gradually and varying the routine sufficiently to challenge all the students and motivate them enough to stay with the program.

What qualifications should an aerobics instructor have?

In the United States there are no laws requiring aerobics instructors to be licensed. However, most athletic clubs and other organizations that sponsor fitness classes require that their teachers be certified.

Two major certifying organizations are the Aerobics and Fitness Association of America (AFAA) in Sherman Oaks, California, and the American Council on Exercise (ACE) in San Diego. Several other national and regional groups also provide certification. Although most qualifying organizations do not require a degree in a fitness-related field, a thorough knowledge of exercise science is needed to pass their examinations (a written one and, in some cases, practical and oral exams as well).

After being certified, most instructors join one of the professional organizations for exercise teachers. These provide regular newsletters, which include information on the latest research studies and choreographic material, and also seminars, conventions, and workshops to help teachers keep up-to-date.

In Canada the Ontario Fitness Council (OFC) and some YMCAs and YWCAs offer certification on satisfactory completion of 60 hours of training.

How do I choose an aerobics class?

The best way to locate a good aerobics class is to ask friends and family members for a recommendation. You can also talk with people who work in local fitness clubs. If you live in a small town, you may have few choices; in a city you will probably find a wealth of classes to choose from.

To find out whether you will feel comfortable with the workout offered and well exercised afterward, observe or participate in a class. Usually you can attend one session without paying in order to decide if a class is for you.

What is the difference between the various intensities of aerobics?

A low-intensity routine is suitable for beginners and anyone recovering from illness or injury. It allows a gradual buildup toward fitness but provides a limited cardiovascular workout. Medium-intensity aerobics improve fitness levels more quickly. High-intensity classes, which usually last longer and include a wider range of activities, are for people striving to bring their fitness to a peak. They are often attended by athletes who are seriously training for another sport.

Some classes are a mixture of low, medium, and high intensity. These may be offered in smaller communities, where numbers of students and available space are too limited to accommodate each level of fitness separately. Such classes can work very well because they allow friends to work out together, even if they have different abilities, and permit people to stay with a favorite instructor as they advance in fitness levels.

A good teacher will interrupt the routine after 20 minutes of aerobic activity to allow students to check their heart rates. If your rate is higher than 85 percent of your maximum, you should slow down. If it is not up to at least 65 percent, you need to work harder (see page 61).

Some people believe that high-impact aerobics—which include a lot of jumping—are the only way to get a high intensity workout. We now know that jumping is not necessary and, in fact, can be very hard on the knee and ankle joints.

Are the steps easy to learn?

At first you may be baffled by the steps and the speed with which they change. Don't worry. After only a few classes you will become familiar with the different movements. Instructors repeat at least some of the steps at every lesson, making it easier to remember them.

What if I find a class too difficult?

Don't be embarrassed to take a break if you need to rest. It is vital to know your limits and be able to judge when you are pushing yourself too hard, or you may put your health at risk. Experienced instructors are familiar with most problems associated with aerobics and will offer you advice and encouragement.

How long will a class last and how will it be structured?

Most sessions last an hour, but some high-intensity classes take up to 2 hours. A class will typically begin with a warm-up and stretches to loosen muscles before going into the aerobic part of the routine, which should last at least 20 minutes. The regimen may also incorporate toning exercises, often in a sequence of 12 exercises, with 2 minutes spent on each one. The class ends with a cooldown routine and stretches, plus deep-breathing exercises to relax you. Afterward you may feel tired or even a little light-headed, but you should feel refreshed and satisfied with your efforts.

What should I wear?

The main criterion for aerobics clothes is that they not restrict your movements; otherwise, it doesn't matter what you wear—a leotard and leggings, a T-shirt and shorts, or a track suit is fine. Wearing layers, such as a sweatshirt over a leotard, is a good idea. You can remove the sweatshirt after warming up and put it back on for the cool-

down period. Well-made footwear is important; shoes should be flexible, with a sole that grips well and extra cushioning (see page 71).

What makes a good instructor?

A good instructor is the key to keeping students motivated and attending on a regular basis. Generally, such a person has a friendly and outgoing personality and encourages participants to enjoy the session while continuing to push their physical limits. He or she will vary the routines and add new elements regularly to prevent the class from becoming boring.

The teacher should arrive well before a class is due to start, to prepare the music, be available to class members who have questions, and consult with new people.

WHAT YOU CAN DO AT HOME

Creating your own music tape for aerobics can be a great way to practice routines at home. Design your tape to last 20 minutes. Most pop songs are 3 to 4 minutes long, so you'll need to select 5 or 6 songs.

Choose music with a basic 4/4 beat (the standard rock/pop rhythm). The tempo, or speed, at which this rhythm is played varies widely; the ideal is between 128 and 135 beats per minute. Select two slightly slower songs for the initial 6 minutes of warm-up. Record the middle 8 minutes from songs with a faster tempo (up to 160 beats per minute for an intense aerobic workout). For the final 6 minutes, choose music once again with a slower tempo to allow your body to cool down gradually as you bring your routine to an end.

EXERCISE CUES
An aerobics instructor uses both visual and verbal cues to prepare the class for a change of movement in plenty of time for participants to make the necessary adjustment.

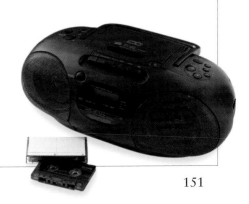

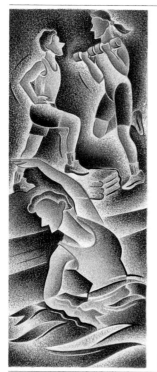

PROS AND CONS OF EXERCISE CLASSES

A variety of exercise classes is available. Each one offers different benefits that may help you better meet your exercise goals as your fitness levels progress; it is well worth taking the time to become familiar with everything that is offered.

TYPES OF CLASSES	ADVANTAGES	DISADVANTAGES
Aerobics	Improve aerobic fitness in an enjoyable social setting.	The movements can be intimidating for those who are not well coordinated.
Step aerobics	Can be high intensity but low impact, thus limiting stress on the joints.	Participants may need several sessions to learn the foot patterns.
Aqua aerobics	Good for pregnant women and anyone with disabilities or joint ailments.	Although swimming ability is not needed, nonswimmers may feel uncomfortable.
Dance aerobics	Provide an enjoyable way to exercise, particularly for those who like dancing.	The movements can be intimidating for those who lack coordination.
Power workout	Ideal for regular exercisers who want a very high-intensity workout.	Not suitable for anyone who is just starting regular aerobics classes.
New body aerobics	Foster aerobic and muscle conditioning.	Not suitable for beginners.
Body sculpting/body toning	Improves muscle tone and strength.	Provides limited aerobic benefits.

warm-up and aerobic sections. The music has a dance tempo, and instructors teach choreographed routines that involve more complex steps than those practiced in standard aerobics classes.

Step aerobics
Originally developed as a form of rehabilitation exercise in Atlanta, Georgia, step aerobics quickly became popular and led to the development of a number of different step routines and home fitness videos. Each participant in a step class has his or her own step platform. The height is usually adjustable according to an individual's fitness level—the higher the step, the harder the workout—and people of all levels work out together. An instructor leads the class in stepping on and off the platform, using a variety of steps and turns. For safety reasons the speed of music used for a step class is usually a little slower than that for a standard or dance aerobics class.

Aqua aerobics
An aqua aerobics class takes place in a swimming pool, ideally in water that reaches to about the middle of the chest. This depth allows the water to support the lower body while providing resistance during the exercises. The instructor stands on the side of the pool so that he or she can supervise and be seen by all participants. An aqua aerobics class follows a format similar to that of a standard aerobics class but is adapted to allow for the slower speed of movement in water.

Power workout
A power workout is an aerobics class that provides a high-intensity regimen for advanced participants. The aerobics section may be high impact and strenuous, possibly lasting up to 50 minutes, so it is advisable to inquire about the level and content of a power workout class before attending.

Body sculpting and toning
The emphasis of a body-sculpting and toning class is on muscular strength and endurance and involves mainly resistance

AEROBICS IN WATER
Because the water supports the body, it eases strain on the joints. Aqua aerobics are therefore ideal for exercisers who are recovering from a back or joint injury. They also provide safe and effective exercise for pregnant women.

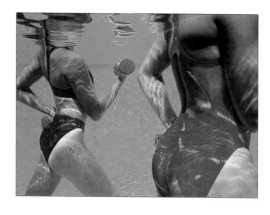

exercises performed to music. Some exercises, such as squats and lunges, may be performed standing, whereas others, like abdominal curls and push-ups, are done on a floor mat. Body-toning classes often incorporate light weight-training equipment, such as rubber bands or ankle weights, to increase the resistance on the muscles.

New body aerobics

New body aerobics, developed originally in Australia, are based on the same format as a regular aerobics class. The participants perform low-impact moves to music during the aerobics section while holding light hand weights. This approach allows the body to develop muscular strength and endurance at the same time that cardiovascular fitness is improving. New body aerobics are a good example of a class that is high in intensity but low in impact.

PLANNING YOUR OWN EXERCISE WORKOUT

To supplement exercise classes, you may want to schedule additional sessions on your own at home or in a gym. When planning your first exercise workout, it is probably best to aim for a session of cardiovascular exercise only, unless you are already quite fit and specifically want to improve your strength or flexibility.

As your confidence and fitness grow, try to add a selection of resistance exercises to your workout. In this way you'll be maximizing your fitness and making the best use

> ### DID YOU KNOW?
> Jane Fonda was the first in a long line of celebrities to appear in an aerobics video in what is now a multimillion-dollar industry. Other stars include Cindy Crawford and Cher. Because of injuries sustained by home exercisers and the resulting legal actions, aerobics video makers now have to make sure that exercises are safe, as well as effective.

of your gym's facilities. Vary the intensity of the workout so that you are training your body to work efficiently at different levels of energy exertion. It is best to keep a balance between the intensity of the different components of your exercise session and the time you take doing them. If the duration increases, the intensity should decrease to avoid premature fatigue. Conversely, if the intensity escalates, the time spent should be reduced. The pyramid system (see below) provides a good way of achieving this.

For an effective cardiovascular routine, the longest time should be spent at the lowest intensity—about 50 percent of training time at levels 1 and 2 (or 65 to 70 percent of maximum heart rate—see "Training Intensity" and table on page 36). As the intensity is increased, the time spent is reduced. The shortest time is spent at the highest levels of intensity—no more than 10 percent at levels 4 and 5, or up to 85 percent of maximum heart rate.

Circuit training

Circuit-training classes consist of a series of exercise stations, some involving a piece of equipment like steps or jump ropes, which are situated at various points around the exercise hall. Participants work their way around the circuit doing exercises at each station in turn. Circuit-training classes start with a warm-up and finish with stretches but otherwise vary greatly. The type of exercises included determines the aerobic and strength-building potential. Circuit training often includes weight-training equipment and so may be held in a gym.

THE PYRAMID SYSTEM

The pyramid system is a structured way of varying training intensity within one workout. In this system the intensity is increased to a predetermined level in gradual stages and then brought back down again in stages.

A typical example is to jog on a treadmill for 5 minutes at a slow speed, for 3 minutes at moderate speed, and then for 1 minute as fast as you can. Slowing the pace, jog for another 2 minutes at roughly between moderate and high speed, 3 minutes at moderate speed, and finally 5 minutes at a slow speed.

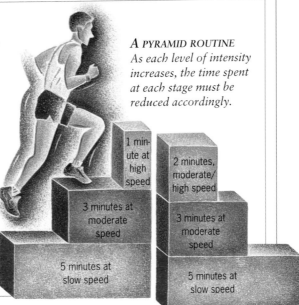

A PYRAMID ROUTINE
As each level of intensity increases, the time spent at each stage must be reduced accordingly.

1 minute at high speed

3 minutes at moderate speed

5 minutes at slow speed

2 minutes, moderate/high speed

3 minutes at moderate speed

5 minutes at slow speed

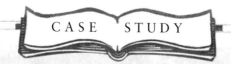

A Menopausal Woman

As a woman's body changes with age, fluctuating hormone levels can cause distressing and debilitating symptoms, from headaches to disturbed sleep and irritability. Add to these problems the pressure of work and low self-esteem, and it can be very difficult to break the cycle of symptoms and depression. A supportive exercise class may provide the solution to some of these difficulties.

Marion is a 52-year-old teacher who has been suffering increasingly troubling menopausal symptoms for nearly a year. She has found that fatigue, irritability, headaches, and hot flashes are keeping her awake at night, affecting her work, and contributing to depression. She feels that she will not be able to face another term at school without help.

Her doctor has advised a course of hormone replacement therapy (HRT), but Marion is nervous about the treatment because friends have told her about side effects they have experienced. However, she feels she may have no choice if her work is not to suffer. She has decided to voice her fears to her doctor and ask for advice on alternatives to HRT.

WHAT SHOULD MARION DO?

Marion's doctor was able to allay many of her fears about HRT but was also willing to suggest certain alternatives, including dietary changes and an exercise program. These may help overcome her symptoms of depression, anxiety, and insomnia and improve her energy levels while also increasing her general well being. Marion found a dietitian who helped her to plan meals. She felt self-conscious about joining a gym because of her age and recent weight gain. A friend introduced her to a gym that runs women-only sessions and has instructors who tailor routines to individuals. These teachers also understand the physical and psychological needs of older women.

Action Plan

HEALTH
Ask a doctor about conventional and alternative treatments for menopause and make sure all questions are answered before rejecting or agreeing to treatment.

EMOTIONAL HEALTH
Find a gym or exercise class that doesn't intimidate her. As Marion gains in confidence, her self-image will improve.

FITNESS
Build up strength, stamina, and suppleness to help relieve symptoms and improve fitness and emotional health.

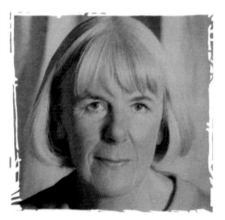

HEALTH
Horror stories from friends or relatives can provoke fear of conventional treatments. Don't dismiss medical help without professional guidance.

EMOTIONAL HEALTH
Age and physical changes, such as weight gain or water retention, can cause self-consciousness and lead to feelings of inadequacy and poor self-image.

FITNESS
Lethargy and general aches and pains may make exercising in public unappealing.

HOW THINGS TURNED OUT FOR MARION

Dietary changes, coupled with mild and carefully monitored medication, helped Marion in the first few weeks, but she felt that long-term relief came from her regular exercise class. At the gym Marion met other women with similar problems and gained support from them. Her symptoms subsided and her fitness improved. She now feels more confident about work, her energy levels are higher, and she is looking forward to the new term.

BEFORE AND AFTER EXERCISE

To get the most from a health club, take advantage of its various facilities to help you prepare for—and recover from—your exercise program.

Taking time to prepare your body and mind before a workout will enhance every aspect of your training and ensure a more effective workout. Physically you will be in the best possible condition—with your body fueled and ready to go—and mentally you will have your mind focused on the task immediately ahead rather than on work or family matters.

Just as conditioning yourself beforehand will set you up for a productive workout, spending time to cool down properly can help your body recover from the increased effort that has been demanded of it. This can be accomplished by stretching all of your muscles thoroughly and then encouraging increased blood flow throughout the body by using various forms of hydrotherapy (see page 156).

BEFORE EXERCISE

About two hours before a session, eat a light, carbohydrate-rich snack; about 50 grams (1¼ ounces) of such foods as dried fruit, whole-grain cereal or crackers, or a bagel with a little jam is ideal. This will allow time for adequate digestion and provide around 200 calories of energy. You should also drink 225 to 300 milliliters (8 to 10 fluid ounces) of water to provide adequate hydration for absorbing and metabolizing the food. You should also have water or fruit juice just before working out. Many health clubs have café or restaurant facilities where you can get a beverage.

It's important to prepare yourself mentally for your session as well. To avoid the anxiety of rushing, allow plenty of time to get to the facility. If you find your mind is preoccupied with work or home problems, set aside five minutes to sit down and unwind before you begin. Meditating or clearing your mind of distracting thoughts will help you to unwind from stresses and pressures. When high levels of stress are prolonged, they can activate potentially damaging hormones, such as cortisol, that can interfere with energy metabolism and inhibit efficient neuromuscular action. These effects in turn can cause such symptoms as lethargy and poor concentration.

If your levels of stress or tension are of particular concern and a short spell of quiet contemplation is not sufficient, you could try a sports massage before your exercise session. This will loosen tight muscles, increase the flow of blood through tissues, relax you, and help counteract the effects of stress hormones.

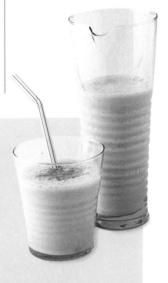

BANANA CINNAMON SMOOTHIE

Many health clubs offer re-energizing snacks and drinks; smoothies are particularly popular because they pack a lot of nutrition into an easily digestible form of food. Here is an energy-boosting recipe you can try at home.

250 ml (9 fl oz) skim or low-fat (1%) milk
115 ml (4 oz) nonfat or low-fat plain yogurt
1 tbsp honey
1 banana, cut in chunks
¼ tsp cinnamon

■ Put all the ingredients in a blender or food processor and blend at high speed for about 10 seconds or until the mixture is smooth.
■ Chill for at least half an hour before serving. Alternatively, pour the mixture into molds and place in the freezer to make a delicious frozen yogurt.
■ Sprinkle extra cinnamon over the top before serving.
Makes two 240-ml (8-ounce) servings.

CREATING A SAUNA EFFECT AT HOME

The benefits of a sauna in relieving sore and tired muscles can be achieved by alternating hot and cold water in your shower (see caution, far right, before proceeding).

▶ *Stand in the shower and run the water as hot as is comfortable until your skin develops a pleasant pink flush.*

▶ *Quickly lower the water temperature to cold (this will cause the blood to be shunted to the core of the body), then run it hot again.*

▶ *You can repeat the process of fluctuating the water temperature as often as desired, but sessions of 30 to 60 seconds are usually sufficient.*

SAUNA RELIEF
Having a sauna after a vigorous workout can help speed the recovery of the muscles.

AFTER EXERCISE

A thorough post-exercise routine, including cooling-down exercises (see page 70) and extra stretches, will improve the suppleness of your muscles and joints and help prevent muscle soreness. An enhanced cool-down might include a 5- to 10-minute swim. This light activity aids blood circulation without placing great stress on the working muscles. Improved circulation encourages the breakdown of any lactic acid that has accumulated in the muscles through anaerobic activity and at the same time helps facilitate the repair of any damage to muscle fibers that might have occurred during the workout.

Hydrotherapy

You can also help cleanse your muscles with hydrotherapy techniques, such as taking a hot bath or shower. The hot water raises the body's temperature and causes the blood to move from the muscles within the body and spread out toward the surface of the skin, giving rise to a pink, flushed appearance. This process is called flushing and is also known as a blood shunt. It is an effective method of getting the blood moving through the worked muscles, thus aiding the removal of lactic acid and other waste products of metabolism.

The effect of the flushing process on the bloodstream is reversed by applying cold water, which causes the blood to be shunted to the core of the body again, thus creating another opportunity to flush waste products out of the muscles. This is what takes place

CAUTION

When alternating hot and cold showers, avoid wetting your head because the temperature fluctuations on the brain can cause dizzy spells or fainting. Anyone who suffers from a heart disorder or high blood pressure should avoid this technique altogether.

during the process of alternating hot and cold showers (see far left column).

If your gym has a sauna, use it after a workout to help your body recuperate. Before entering it, take an initial cleansing shower, running the water down to a cold temperature. When you enter the sauna, sit down on the lowest, or coolest, level until you have acclimatized to the high temperature. After 5 to 10 minutes, move to a higher position to raise the body temperature. Do not spend more than 15 minutes at a time in a sauna because doing so can cause the body to overheat.

When you leave the sauna, take a cold shower for one to two minutes, then return to the cool area of the sauna for two more minutes to assist flushing. In most clubs this is considered a single use of the sauna; up to five visits to the sauna will be enough to assist your recuperation.

Muscle soreness

If any symptoms of muscle soreness appear in the days following a workout, the best remedy, in addition to the self-help techniques described on page 148, is to make the muscles lightly perform activities that are similar to the exercise movements used in the workout that led to the soreness. This ensures that the sore muscles are being flushed with blood to assist recovery.

The intensity of such activity must be kept below the threshold of aerobic work, or it will generate more muscle fatigue and potential soreness. Between 55 and 65 percent of your maximum heart rate (see page 61) is considered the ideal level at which to work. This strategy, called active recovery, is far more effective than just resting and doing nothing after exercise, which is known as passive recovery. Active recovery can dissipate muscular soreness in less than half the time needed for passive recovery.

INDEX

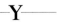

ACKNOWLEDGMENTS

Carroll & Brown Limited
would like to thank
Budo Store
Chartered Society of Physiotherapists
Chartered Society of Sports
    Physiotherapists
Hales Sports Shop
Holmes Place Health and Fitness Club
Obesity Resource Information Centre
Porcelli Dance Shop
Sports Council
Malcolm Whyatt, Oscar Heidenstam
    Foundation

Editorial assistance
Sharon Freed
Jennifer Mussett
Nadia Silver
Simon Warmer

Design assistance
Evie Loizides
Gilda Pacitti

DTP design
Elisa Merino

Photograph sources
9 (Top) Hulton Getty Picture
    Collection
10 (Top) Hulton Getty Picture
    Collection
11 (Top) Tony Stone Images
16 Juan Alvarez/Image bank
19 *and front cover* (Bottom left)
    Angela Hampton/Family Life
    Pictures
21 (Top) CNRI/SPL;
    (Bottom) All Action
22 (Top) The Post Office
23 Museum of Fine Arts/Bridgeman
    Art Library
28 (Bottom) Sporting Pictures UK
    Ltd

33 (Left, centre and bottom)
    Sporting Pictures UK Ltd
34 The Stock Market
35 Sporting Pictures UK Ltd
36 (Left) Rex Features
39 The Stock Market
41 The Stock Market
42 Robert Harding Picture Library
45 Alain Deniz/Frank Spooner
    Pictures
53 Will and Deni McIntyre/SPL
60 Larry J. Pierce/Image Bank
64 Mary Evans Picture Library
67 (Top) Sporting Pictures UK Ltd
73 Rex Features
78 (Top) Philips Domestic
    Appliance and Personal Care
81 (Top) SPL; (Bottom) John
    Greim/SPL
82 (Top) D. Mossiat/Frank Spooner
    Pictures; (Bottom) The Dame
    Rosalind Paget Trust
84 (Bottom) The Stock Market
86 The Stock Market
89 The Stock Market
92 (Top) Tony Stone Images
93 Collections/Anthea Sieveking
95 (Left) Rex features; (Centre and
    right) Sporting Pictures UK Ltd
96 (Top) Rex Features
97 (Top) Popperfoto
98 (Top) Angela Hampton/Family
    Life Pictures
100 (Top) Telegraph Colour Library;
    (Bottom) Rex Features
102 Telegraph Colour Library
103 (Right) Tony Stone
104 Sporting Pictures UK Ltd
105 (Top) Brylak/Frank Spooner
    Pictures
106 (Top) The Hutchison Library
107 (Top) Tony Stone Images
108 (Top) The Telegraph Colour
    Library
109 Rex Features
110 (Top) Tony Stone Images
111 (Top) Rex Features

112 (Top) Rex Features
114 (Top left) The Telegraph Colour
    Library; (Right) Rex Features
115 (Top) Rex Features
116 Simon Grosset/Frank Spooner
    Pictures
117 (Top and bottom left) The
    Stock Market
118 (Top) Rex Features
120 The Stock Market
132 Telegraph Colour Library
136 Mary Evans Picture Library
138 The Stock Market
141 The Oscar Heidenstam
    Foundation
150 (Bottom) Corbis-Bettman/UPI
152 Tony Stone Images
156 The Stock Market

Illustrators
Debbie Hinks
Conny Jude
Alan Nanson
David Stevens
Josephine Sumner
Paul Williams

Photographic assistant
Mark Langridge

Hair and make-up
Kim Menzies
Jessamina Owens

Picture research
Sandra Schneider

Food preparation
Maddalena Bastianelli

Research
Steven Chong

Index
Richard Emerson

75-010-02